King
Cancer

King Cancer

The Good, the Bad and the Cure of Cancer

by

Philip Nobile

Sheed and Ward, Inc.
Subsidiary of Universal Press Syndicate
New York

Library of Congress Catalog Card Number 74-10162
ISBN: 0-8362-0544-8

To my dear mother
MARGARET NOBILE
1917-1972
who died nobly of cancer

Contents

Acknowledgments

A journalist is only as good as his sources. It was my good fortune to make the acquaintance and receive the hospitality of many cancer experts. Without their unbounded cooperation I could not have written this book.

I would like to cite the following sources for a special degree of assistance: Dr. Michael Hanna of Oak Ridge National Laboratory in Oak Ridge, Tennessee; Dr. Jerome Urban, Dr. Robin Watson, and Dr. William G. Cahan of Memorial Sloan-Kettering Hospital in New York City; Dr. Sidney Cutler of the National Cancer Institute in Bethesda, Maryland; Dr. Albert Owens of Johns Hopkins Hospital in Baltimore; Dr. Edward Reich of Rockefeller University, New York City; Dr. Edmund Klein of Roswell Park Memorial Institute in Buffalo; Arthur Godfrey; Ed McCaskey of the Chicago Bears; Benno Schmidt, chairman of the President's Cancer Panel; and Dr. James Watson of Harvard University.

Dr. Frank Rauscher, director of the National Cancer Institute, graciously opened the doors of NCI to me; NCI Director of Public Affairs Frank Karel and his assistant Mrs. Alice Hamm were of immense help.

Dr. William Beattie, chief medical officer of Memorial Sloan-Kettering Hospital, kindly allowed me total access to his institution.

I greatly appreciate the perception of my Sheed and Ward editor, Donna Martin.

Judy Greenwald, formerly a reporter at *Medical World News,* helped with the research as I expanded my *Esquire* article (also entitled "King Cancer") into this book.

But most of all I want to recognize a debt to Tom Ferrell, managing editor of *Esquire* and a friend, who first asked me to write about cancer and guided the original manuscript with great care and intelligence.

Preface

Cancer is the disease to end diseases. It is painful, disfiguring, debilitating, costly and usually fatal. Treatment is especially rough. And strangest of all, the cure is measured in survival time! According to the American Cancer Society, a cancer victim is pronounced "cured" if there is no "evidence of the disease at least five years after diagnosis and treatment."

That's some kind of cure. Actually, the original cancer can recur in the sixth year or the twentieth year. Two-thirds of all cancer victims are dead within five years. Yet most of the remaining one-third, the allegedly cured, will also die from their tumors.

Progress is exceedingly slow. Since 1930, the size of the survival group has increased only 13 percentage points. For example, forty-five years ago only 20 percent of cancer patients survived five years as opposed to 33 percent who survive today. Depending on your point of view, this increase is cause for great optimism pointing toward inevitable victory or steady pessimism emphasizing the ultimate intractibility of the disease.

Cancer specialists are professional optimists. They are prone to see light at the end of their tunnel. Other medicine men simply throw up their hands in the face of malignancy. Cancer is curable, they admit, but not by presently known and practiced means. This book reflects the tug of war between the optimists and the pessimists as well as the intramural conflict among the optimists themselves. For even those specialists who believe cancer is curable violently disagree on procedure.

It is a disease to end diseases, is it not?

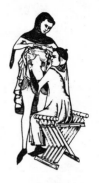

CHAPTER ONE

The Day They
Cured Cancer

On Friday evening, September 22, 1972, Dr. Michael
Hanna was paged three times during a showing of *A
Clockwork Orange* at the Ridge Theater in Oak
Ridge, Tennessee. He took each call in the closed box
office outside, where he was distracted by late arrivals
who insisted on buying tickets. After the third inter-
ruption, he told the manager to say he had left. The
calls were making him nervous and, besides, he didn't
want to miss any more of "the old in-and-out"
scenes. Hanna is a doctor of zoology, not medicine.

1

He had every right to turn off at the movies, but not that night, not since he had just "cured" cancer.

UPI rushed the miraculous news—rated "UR-GENT"—over its national wire about 8 P.M. Eastern Standard Time:

> Scientists say they have found a bacterial agent that is "100 percent effective" against cancer in animals and will soon begin full-fledged testing on humans.
>
> Dr. Michael Hanna, Jr., head of immunology at the Oak Ridge National Laboratory, said today some limited, preliminary testing on humans has been done with the agent, called BCG, in California and France. He said scientists may begin treating patients with BCG within a few months.
>
> "It has been 100 percent effective in animals. And in humans, in the cases done, it is good enough to say that it is the most encouraging thing to come along in a long time."

While Hanna sat apprehensively incommunicado, radio and TV stations all over the country were desperately trying to make contact. Morning newspapers were already setting the story in type. The *Detroit News* would run it on the front page with the headline "New Cancer Treatment Revealed"; The *Washington Star*, more optimistic, went with "New Find Raises Hope of Real Cancer Cures." Another *War of the Worlds* incident was passing beyond the fail-safe point, and cancer victims and their families would soon be getting "the old in-and-out" themselves.

Hanna knew something was wrong. Reporters had

never telephoned him at the movies before. And what was it one of them mentioned about a "cure for cancer" on the UPI wire? He couldn't fathom it. Earlier in the day he had talked briefly with Carl Vine, UPI's veteran Knoxville correspondent, about a BCG experiment on guinea pigs he had recently completed in conjunction with two National Cancer Institute scientists. Vine rang him up after reading an NCI handout on the team's work in that afternoon's *Knoxville News Sentinel*. He thought there might be a local-interest angle in the story, probably worth a couple of paragraphs in some eastern Tennessee papers. BCG was nothing earth-shattering to Vine. He covered an immunology conference at Gatlinburg, Tennessee, back in May and interviewed all the important BCG people then.

Bacillus Calmette-Guerin (BCG)—a strain of tuberculosis bacteria used as an anti-TB vaccine in Europe—has been bumping around cancer research for years with variable clinical results. The basic theory is quite simple: when BCG is introduced into the body (animal or human), the body's immune system recognizes it as foreign and goes in for the kill with an armada of freshly recruited white cells. Sometimes this same immune reaction is lethal for foreign cancer cells as well. At Gatlinburg, for example, Dr. Edmund Klein of Buffalo's Roswell Park Memorial Institute reported five cases of remission in inoperable breast cancers after treatments with a BCG-like salve.

Hanna told Vine that his experiment showed that

injections of BCG into transplanted skin tumors of guinea pigs not only destroyed the tumor but also caught the spreading cancer in the lymph nodes. This reaction occurred in every guinea pig tested. Shortly after six o'clock, Vine filed a straightforward three hundred word story over UPI's local wire.

The dispatch was read in UPI's state office in Nashville and at the service's southern headquarters in Atlanta. Both places were intrigued and decided the story needed some buildup. Vine had retired for the evening, so the job fell to Nashville's Janell Glasgow, the only UPI reporter on duty that Friday night. "I was it for the state of Tennessee," she comments, "and Atlanta was having a fit. Well, I was sitting there trying to figure out why they were calling me back every five minutes. I assumed it was a nice, normal story and frankly I didn't see much in it. But New York was pressing Atlanta and they told me to just do it."

She reached Hanna at home around seven and took the troublesome "100 percent effective in animals" quote down on her typewriter. Then she fed her material to Atlanta, where the final flourishes were executed. Atlanta wired the story to New York for a national sendoff and the rest is history. "What I wonder in this whole mishmash," remarks the twenty-seven-year-old Glasgow, who is no longer with UPI, "is whether a science reporter ever got a look at the copy. You say you have a liberal arts degree and UPI loves you."

According to UPI's Atlanta news editor, Bruce Bakke, no science person saw the story there. "We have a science editor," admits Bill Laffler, General Desk news editor at UPI in New York, "but he's a victim of cancer himself and hasn't been in for a year. Ordinarily we would have checked the story out with him, especially one that raises people's hopes." (The UPI editor in question subsequently died.)

Saturday the predictable happened. If BCG, as UPI declared, was universally curing cancer in animals and would soon be tested in humans, then naturally every cancer patient would covet a supply for himself. Phone calls poured into medical centers in every state begging for injections. Mercy flights to Oak Ridge were readied by anxious families. Car caravans headed for Hanna's home. A man from Australia wanted to fly over his sick horse. In a macabre twist, half the messages left for Hanna were from people with dying pets. Hanna retreated to his Oak Ridge lab where he sensed things closing in. "I didn't feel bad for myself, but for those people. It made me realize we were playing for keeps."

Meanwhile Dr. Herbert J. Rapp, the NCI immunologist who designed the guinea pig model for Hanna, was boiling. His ten-year project, which Hanna had only recently joined, seemed to be slipping away from him. The proper allotment of glory concerned him more than the tragedies being played out on BCG weekend. He felt bad that the national publicity was sailing along without him. "If there were any credit to be gained from all this Mike would be getting it," lamented Rapp.

The original NCI release in the Knoxville paper had been Rapp's own doing. He wanted some attention for his joint experiment with Hanna and NCI colleague Berton Zbar. Rapp edited the language himself. In its pristine form, the BCG story appeared innocuous. Clearly, the experiment was limited to guinea pigs. There was no indication of "100 percent" effectiveness, although the first sentence included the phrase "complete disappearance." True enough. Each guinea pig tested experienced a "complete disappearance" of its tumor. Rapp might have specified that the experiment pertained solely to skin tumors, but nonetheless the key was low and no suggestion of breakthrough was implied. If Hanna ever really said (and he's not sure he did) that BCG was "100 percent effective in animals," he meant *only* in his laboratory guinea pigs and *only* with tumors transplanted into their breasts. That was the context of his remark. But nobody in the UPI chain saw fit to question what proved to be a disastrously misleading quotation, or to check it with someone other than Hanna.

Frank Karel, NCI public affairs director, believes the Rapp-approved release was defective. Rapp resents this charge. "The release is factual," he insists. "What more do you want? Karel's not qualified to comment, scientifically or any other way. And by the way, they're increasing the publicity department at NCI at the expense of research."

In order to cool the BCG crisis, NCI had to put out a clarifying statement. Rapp wrote his own version, which was promptly killed by Dr. Bayard H. Morrison, assistant director of NCI. Morrison was after something more critical and he got it. The icy clarification, issued the next Wednesday, left little doubt that NCI was shipping BCG out to sea. "There's a faction here that doesn't want immunology to succeed," Rapp claims. "They honestly don't think it can succeed. So they act accordingly. Their statement is calculated to shove BCG under the rug. But BCG isn't going away, it's going to snowball."

Someone close to the BCG research project surveyed the dispute and laughed disgustedly. "If I came up with a cure for cancer tomorrow, half the people at the National Cancer Institute would commit suicide and the other half would be out chasing me with a machine gun. The jealousy is so great."

Welcome to the conquest of cancer.

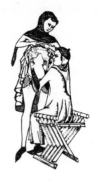

CHAPTER TWO

First The Bad News, Then The Good

(1) *The Bad News*

Cancer is the leading cause of death in the United States except for diseases of the heart. It kills more women between thirty and fifty-four than any other factor and more children under fifteen than any other disease (nearly 3,500 childhood deaths are predicted for 1975). After accidents, cancer racks up the highest mortality rate in people under thirty-five. And that's just for openers.

It is estimated that four out of five Americans who get cancer will die of it sooner or later no matter how early the diagnosis or vigorous the treatment. At current rates of incidence, cancer will strike one quarter of the population and approximately two out of every three families. In 1975, approximately 1,000

Mortality for Leading Causes of Death: United States, 1971

Rank	Cause of Death	Number of Deaths	Death Rate Per 100,000 Population	Percent of Total Deaths
	All Causes	1,927,542	932.2	100.0
1	Diseases of Heart	743,138	359.5	38.6
2	Cancer	337,398	163.2	17.5
3	Stroke	209,092	101.1	10.8
4	Accidents	113,439	54.9	5.9
5	Influenza & Pneumonia	57,194	27.7	3.0
6	Certain Diseases of Infancy	38,494	18.6	2.0
7	Diabetes Mellitus	38,256	18.5	2.0
8	Cirrhosis of Liver	31,808	15.4	1.7
9	Arteriosclerosis	31,521	15.2	1.6
10	Suicide	24,092	11.7	1.2
11	Emphysema	22,539	10.9	1.2
12	Homicide	18,787	9.1	1.0
13	Congenital Anomalies	15,957	7.7	0.8
14	Nephritis and Nephrosis	8,443	4.1	0.4
15	Hypertension	7,837	3.8	0.4
	Other & Ill-Defined	229,547	110.8	11.9

Source: Vital Statistics of the United States, 1971
Prepared by: Research Department, American Cancer Society, July, 1974

Americans a day will drop off from cancer, 655,000 new cases will be spotted for the first time (not including superficial skin cancer and carcinoma-in-situ of the uterine cervix), and 1,025,000 will be under medical care for cancer. The annual direct and indirect cost of all this sickness and death is over $15 billion.

Cancer among males increased 50 percent between 1936 and the present, with black males showing a distinctly dramatic gain. Lung cancer is now epidemic—the mortality rate went up 2000 percent for men in the past forty years and women's rates are rising even faster. It is second in incidence only to colon-rectum cancer overall, and first in incidence in men. Yet, in the ten years since the publication of the Surgeon General's Report on Smoking and Health—which linked cigarettes to cancer—the number of smokers has risen from 50 to 52 million.

Despite advances in detection and surgery, the mortality rate for breast cancer has remained steady for the past thirty-five years.

The five-year relative survival or "cure" rate for all cancers is only 39 percent. Some types are particularly frightening. For example, the five-year relative survival rate for cancer of the pancreas is 1 percent, for the liver and esophagus 3 percent, for the gall bladder 7 percent, for the lung and bronchus 8 percent. and for the stomach 12 percent.

Outside of a few major cancer centers, both the diagnosis and treatment of cancer are risky proposi-

FIVE YEAR CANCER SURVIVAL RATES*
FOR SELECTED SITES

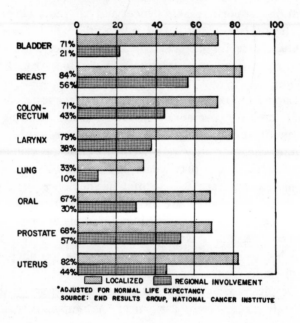

LOCALIZED   REGIONAL INVOLVEMENT

*ADJUSTED FOR NORMAL LIFE EXPECTANCY
SOURCE: END RESULTS GROUP, NATIONAL CANCER INSTITUTE

tions. Historically, the best medical minds have avoided the malady as if it were contagious. The study of cancer is an insignificant part of the medical school curriculum.

Clinical advances are not disseminated widely or rapidly. Only 20 to 25 percent of children with leukemia have access to the best treatment because the latest information hasn't reached the doctors. The left hand often doesn't know what the right hand is doing: voice boxes have been removed unnecessarily by surgeons who didn't know (or care) that radiation was sometimes just as good for cancer of the larynx.

According to the World Health Organization, 75 to 85 percent of all cancers originate in the environment. Industrial chemicals are the principal carcinogenic suspects, but only 450 of the 30,000 compounds are government-regulated.

The Environmental Protection Agency recently revealed that pollutants associated with cancer have been discovered in the water supplies of major cities like Washington, D.C., New Orleans, and Cincinnati.

The American Cancer Society regretfully informs us that: "Some 111,000 1975 cancer patients will die who might have been saved by earlier diagnosis and better treatment." Forty percent of American women in years of peak risk have never had a Pap smear; consequently twelve thousand women die needlessly of cancer of the cervix each year. Only 18 percent of women and 17 percent of men have had a proctoscopic examination, which is crucial to the early detection and cure of colon-rectum cancer, the Number 2 cancer killer in both men (after lung) and women (after breast).

Drugs can be curative (more or less) for about 15 percent of cancers but their side effects include nausea, diarrhea, cirrhosis, oral ulcers, feminization, masculinization, fluid retention, and depression.

Billions have been spent on cancer research since 1937 and its prevention is still a mystery.

Upon the passage of the $1.6 billion National Can-

cer Act of 1971, President Nixon said: "I am determined that the Federal will and Federal resources will
be committed as effectively as possible to the campaign against cancer and that nothing will be allowed
to compromise that commitment." Yet the Nixon
budget for fiscal 1974 shortchanged the congressional
appropriations for the National Cancer Institute to
the tune of $100 million. In the previous two years of
the National Cancer Act authorization, the administration shaved congressional appropriations by $90
million.

Dr. Robert A. Good, director of Memorial Sloan-
Kettering Cancer Center in New York City and formerly a member of the three-man President's Cancer
Panel, said the National Cancer Program is "suffering" from lack of funds.

But there are some cancer specialists who think the
country has been sold a bill of goods on talk about a
quick cure through massive federal aid. "Despite the
concepts and research tools that twenty-five years of
research have developed," insists Nobel Laureate, Dr.
Salvador E. Luria, who is heading up MIT's new
cancer center, "cancer research is not ready for a
crash program approach." Dr. Sol Spiegelman, director of Columbia's Institute of Cancer Research, em-
phasizes that "an all-out effort at this time would be
like trying to land a man on the moon without
knowing Newton's laws of gravity."

Damned if you don't, damned if you do.

And did you hear the one about Dr. Irving Kessler

of Johns Hopkins who tried to prove that you can catch leukemia from household pets?

(2) *The Good News*

Cancer is primarily a disease of old age. More than half of all cancer deaths occur in persons over sixty-five, more than three-quarters over fifty. Although certain cancers run in families and although some environmentally-caused malignancies may be transferred from one family member to another, the disease is not, strictly speaking, hereditary or catching. Leukemia is responsible for half the cancer cases of American children, but happily it is extremely rare (4 per 100,000). The average pediatrician will see only three leukemia sufferers in a lifetime. Presently there are about 1.5 million Americans who have been "cured" of cancer, that is, they are disease-free five years after diagnosis and treatment.

In situ cancer is nearly 100 percent curable. The relative five-year survival rate for localized cancer—that is, cancer which has not started to migrate much beyond its place of origin—is an encouraging 67 percent (as opposed to 39 percent for all stages combined). Cancers of the skin, lip, eye, salivary gland, and thyroid gland have five-year relative survival rates of better than 80 percent.

The cancer death rate has been gradually declining among American women—down 13 percent since 1936—largely due to a sharp reduction in mortality

Cancer Incidence by Site and Sex*

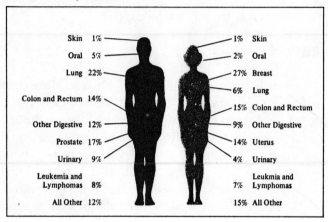

*Excluding superficial skin cancer and carcinoma in situ of uterine cervix.
From '*75 Cancer Facts & Figures* (American Cancer Society)

from cancer of the uterine cervix, a readily detectable disease. In general, the cancer mortality is leveling off except for a few kinds (lung, ovary, pancreas, and leukemia). Stomach cancer death rates have fallen about 50 percent in both sexes in the last twenty years for reasons unknown.

American Indians have markedly less cancer mortality than their white brothers. And so do Eskimos—Alaska claims the lowest per capita cancer death rate of any state in the Union. Utah comes in second with its large population of clean-living, nonsmoking Mormons.

When you come right down to it, cancer deaths are to a large degree preventable—between 30 and 90

Cancer Deaths by Site and Sex

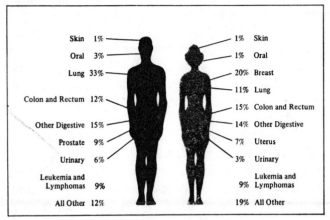

From '75 *Cancer Facts & Figures* (American Cancer Society)

percent preventable according to NCI Director Dr. Frank J. Rauscher, Jr. For example, lung cancer mortality would be reduced 90 percent with the elimination of smoking. Annual proctoscopic examinations of the rectum could cancel out up to three-quarters of the 49,000 colon-rectum cancer deaths a year. Most skin cancers could be prevented by avoiding overexposure to direct sunlight. Pap smears have reduced uterine cancer deaths 65 percent in the past thirty-five years. An early detection method for analyzing cells in the sputum of heavy smokers and certain industrial workers could lead to a substantial decrease in lung cancer mortality. Also certain cancers caused by occupational factors—particularly bladder cancer in the dye industry—have been prevented by eliminating the causative agents.

The National Cancer Act of 1971 provided for the establishment of eighteen new comprehensive cancer centers whose purpose is to foster "the most up-to-date patient care facilities for clinical research and teaching in order to develop and demonstrate the best methods of cancer prevention, diagnosis, treatment, and rehabilitation" (National Cancer Program, *Report of the Director,* January, 1973,). These new model comprehensive cancer center programs are intended to deliver complete geographic coverage. An estimated half of the U.S. population should be within driving distance of the facilities.

In 1974, the American Cancer Society and the National Cancer Institute set up twenty-seven breast-

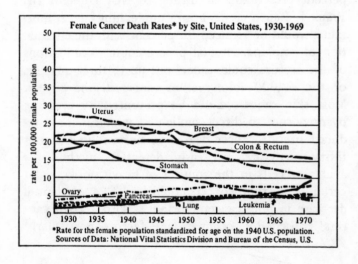

Female Cancer Death Rates* by Site, United States, 1930-1969

*Rate for the female population standardized for age on the 1940 U.S. population.
Sources of Data: National Vital Statistics Division and Bureau of the Census, U.S.

cancer detection centers around the country. Each offers a combination of advanced diagnostic tests and clinical examinations to women over thirty-five, who are without symptoms of breast malignancy. And all examinations are free! And if worse comes to worst, in the opinion of Dr. George Crile, Jr., of the Cleveland Clinic, women need never have a radical mastectomy since "lesser procedures are just as effective."

Despite the party line on cigarettes, otherwise known as cancer sticks, 95 percent of heavy smokers never run afoul of cancer. Although the British Royal College of Physicians declared, "Cigarette smoking is now as important a cause of death as were the great epidemic diseases such as typhoid, cholera, and tuberculosis," a careful British report showed that the chances of smokers dying of lung cancer is only one

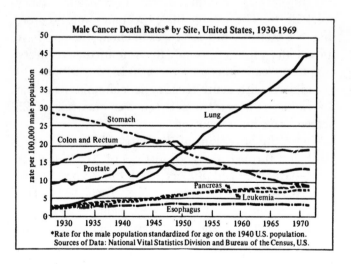

Male Cancer Death Rates* by Site, United States, 1930-1969

*Rate for the male population standardized for age on the 1940 U.S. population.
Sources of Data: National Vital Statistics Division and Bureau of the Census, U.S.

in five hundred. For those who prefer better odds, filter cigarettes may be the answer. Dr. William G. Cahan, a Memorial Sloan-Kettering lung surgeon, expects a better cigarette will make a noticeable difference in future lung mortality statistics. He also argues, contrary to popular assumption, that nicotine is not addictive. And 10 million people have given up smoking the past ten years.

In the cold war against cancer, the United States is burying Russia. "We're several giant steps, many giant steps well ahead," says NCI's Rauscher.

Hodgkins disease, a formerly lethal cancer of the lymph nodes, can now be cured about 90 percent of the time in its early stages with supervoltage x-radiation, and 50 percent of the time in its later stages with a four-drug combination treatment.

Ten years ago childhood leukemia meant a fairly quick death. The average life expectancy was no more than six months. But advances in chemotherapy have turned the picture around. In some medical centers, long-term remissions are now possible for 90 percent of children with acute leucocytic leukemia. Five-year survivals of 50 percent and ten-year survivals of 25 percent have been reported.

Under the provisions of the National Cancer Act of 1971 and through the good offices of Nixon's Office of Management and Budget, $1.3 billion has flowed into NCI's cancer program through fiscal 1974. This three-year outlay (1972–74) exceeded NCI's combined budget for the seven years previous to the National Cancer Act.

The American Cancer Society, a voluntary organization of about 2.3 million citizens and the perennial good guy in the long, once hidden, war on cancer, has dispensed $350 million in its history. Twenty-seven million ACS dollars went into research grants in 1974.

Dr. A. Hamblin Letton, a former president of the American Cancer Society, called the National Cancer Act "probably the greatest thing that has ever been done by the United States."

Many cancer experts insist that the time is ripe for major breakthroughs. Dr. Jonathan E. Rhoads, chairman of the Department of Surgery at the University of Pennsylvania, compares the present state of cancer research to that of atom bomb research in 1939.

The late Dr. Sidney Farber, former director of Research at the Children's Cancer Research Foundation in Boston, felt the moment might be near. "Based on the insights with which I am familiar," he testified before Congress in 1971, "there is no question in my mind that, if we make this effort today, we will in a relatively short period of time make vast inroads on the cancer problem as we know it today leading to the eventual control of cancer."

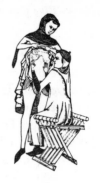

CHAPTER THREE

The Insatiable Monster

The Eternal Watchmaker could not have been Himself the day He created cancer. On the whole, this disease is probably His worst mistake. It comes in over a hundred devastating varieties, each seemingly designed for maximum feasible discomfort. No earthly reason requires cancer to be as ubiquitous as it is invincible. Heart ailments are no joke, but at least they share the advantage of being localized. You can't get a heart attack in the bladder or on the brain. Nor do heart attacks spread to other parts of the body.

But cancer, if it wants you badly enough, and it does, can get you almost anywhere. Name the organ or tissue and cancer is sure to have a customized tumor. However, the true spice of malignancy is not variety, but metastasis. Tumor cells are like subcutaneous greased pigs. They slip and slide (or metastasize) from the surest hands. Once you have had your tumor removed, there's no guarantee that some malignant cells haven't already emigrated to God knows where. And so the death watch begins. You wait for another lump. You pray for continued remission. But more often than not cancer has made you an unbreakable appointment in Samarra.

West Virginia Senator Matthew M. Neely accused cancer of crimes against humanity in a speech on the Senate floor in 1928. His emotional plea has not lost its force:

> I propose to speak of a monster that is more insatiable than the guillotine; more destructive to life and health and happiness than the World War, more irresistible than the mightiest army that ever marched to battle; more terrifying than any scourge that has ever threatened the existence of the human race. The monster of which I speak has infested and still infests every inhabited country; it has preyed and still preys upon every nation; it has fed and feasted and fattened . . . on the flesh and blood and brains and bones of men and women and children in every land. The sighs and sobs and shrieks that it has exhorted from perishing humanity would, if they were tangible things, make a mountain. The tears

that it has wrung from weeping women's eyes would make an ocean. The blood that it has shed would redden every wave that rolls on every sea. The name of this loathsome, deadly and insatiate monster is "cancer."

Although the organized battle against cancer didn't pick up steam until Senator Neely's time (he was the first to push for cancer legislation), the malady had been around for thousands of years. The doctors of Egypt described symptoms and treatment on papyrus. Hippocrates identified several forms and gave cancer its name—*karkinos*—the Greek word for crab, whose claws were compared to the veins that often shoot out from tumors. But in ancient, and even not-so-ancient times, cancer was a comparatively rare disease. According to nineteenth-century French statistics, cancer accounted for only 1.6 percent of all deaths in Paris in 1830. Ten years later the figure rose to 2.4 percent. In the United States today cancer causes 17.5 percent of all mortality, and the figures are even higher in many European countries. Obviously, some of the historical increase can be explained by improvements in life expectancy, diagnostic techniques, and record-keeping. But the principal villain is our growing carcinogenic environment.

Cancer is the by-product of civilization and industrialization. Eight out of ten cancers originate from extrinsic sources. One thousand chemicals have already been found to cause cancer in animals and most of them are still available for human ingestion. New potential carcinogens are brought to us daily through air pollution, food additives, pesticides, and so on.

The incidence of certain cancers fluctuates from country to country. America is big in breast, lung, and colon cancer, but Japan is exceedingly low in these types. However, our stomach rates are way down and theirs are sky high. Different diets are the probable factors here because Japanese-Americans, either immigrants or native-born, tend to approximate U.S. stomach cancer rates and not Japan's. Which food is better for your health—American or Japanese? That depends on whether you prefer cancer in your colon or your stomach.

Africa is relatively free from our civilized malignancies, but the continent has not been forgotten. Burkitt's lymphoma, an ugly facial cancer in children, is endemic in parts of East and South Africa. Eskimos, a fairly resistant race, get cancer in the mouth, perhaps from biting their ash-sprinkled shoe leather into place.

One of the more sinister attributes of cancer is its delayed effect. You never know when you are handing it an invitation. Until the first hooked generation of three-pack-a-day-for-twenty-years smokers came along in the fifties, lung cancer was inconsequential. In 1956, a joint British-American committee studying the effects of radiation on man recommended against indiscriminate exposure to diagnostic X-rays. Pregnant women and children were frequent radiation targets and leukemia was the suspected result—especially since an alarming population of leukemics had just emerged from among the A-bomb victims of Hiroshima and Nagasaki. Doctors and X-ray technicians apparently heeded the committee's advice. For in the sixties there were one thousand fewer deaths from leukemia than had been expected from earlier rates.

A hundred-plus varieties, metastasis, discomfort, suspense, universality, covertness: the monster is loathsome, deadly, and insatiate.

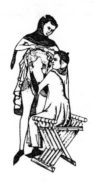

CHAPTER FOUR

An Inside Job

Cancer is the ultimate inside job. It starts conspiratorially within the cell, unseen and unannounced. No discrete triggering particle has yet been linked to human malignancy. No chemical or bug has been observed that automatically turns the normal cell into a microscopic Frankenstein monster. Rather, the genesis of this disease involves immensely complicated, though quite basic, molecular processes. Without cell division, for instance, there would be no cancer. But without cell division, there would also be no life.

Cells must divide—you can't fight evolution. How they do it, though, makes all the difference. Unfortunately, the internal control mechanisms that spell normal or cancerous division are presently beyond biological reach. We simply do not know why mammalian cells continue or stop dividing.

Back to Biology I for a moment: Every cell contains a set of genes—units of hereditary material arranged along chromosomes and constituted of DNA (deoxyribonucleic acid). The chemical DNA through its carrier RNA (ribonucleic acid) determines identity and directs traffic—it tells the embryonic cell what kind of cell it is and where it should go. Liver cells to the liver, bladder cells to the bladder. This process is called differentiation. If all goes well, the differentiated cells (now grouped in various tissues of the body) will replicate themselves in an orderly fashion—at the right time, place, and speed according to the mysterious gene control mechanism. The number of new arrivals should correspond to the number of the deceased. Perfectly balanced cells are healthy cells.

However, the slightest molecular hitch may throw off this delicate equilibrium and tilt the organism in favor of cancer. Four factors seem to influence the synthesis of DNA and therefore the cell's pattern of proliferation. A foul-up can occur in (1) the cytoplasm, the living matter of the cell; (2) the intercellular controls whereby neighboring cells communicate with each other; (3) the hormones which regulate cellular metabolism and gene expression; and (4) the

DNA itself or its messenger RNA, which can be upset by the actions of viruses, chemicals, or radiation. Once DNA is compromised, the genes don't function correctly and the previous normal cell gives birth to a malignant one. Cancer debuts.

Cancer cells have two destructive talents—unlimited growth and metastasis. If the former doesn't suffice to kill the victim, the latter will. When a normal cell divides, only one offspring redivides. But when a cancer cell divides, both offspring do likewise. It is an unrestrained growth of cells, building up into masses or tumors that invade and destroy surrounding tissue. And almost all types of normal cells can be transformed into malignant cells. Such anarchic and invasive expansion contrasts with the "contact inhibition" of the normal cell, which prevents cellular crowding by restricting cell growth to a single layer. The surface of the cancer cell is also less adhesive than that of its normal counterpart. It has no affinity for the primary tumor and so it can migrate to other parts of the body through the bloodstream and lymphatic system. Whenever it stops, it settles and grows. This secondary type of growth is a metastasis. If cancer didn't metastasize, it would be a local or regional affair and hardly the systemic menace it so often is.

Cancer can pop up just about anywhere, although it appears to favor sites where there's a pretty fast turnover in cells—the skin, the lungs, the glands of the breast, the gastrointestinal tract, the blood-forming organs, and the lymphoid tissues. Metastasis has no particular logic. Neighboring organs and lymph nodes are likely locations for a spreading malignancy, but a tumor often metastasizes to distant locations—for example, from the lung to the brain. And the bigger the tumor, the better the chance for metastasis.

Cancer growth is measured according to doubling time, that is, the time it takes for a tumor to double its size. For example, the doubling time for breast cancer is usually between thirty and two hundred days. The variability of this rate explains why breast tumors often seem to be missed at one examination only to be caught in another a few months later. It can be speculated Betty Ford's tumor had a doubling time on the far end of the spectrum because a previous breast examination showed no evidence of malignancy just seven months earlier.

There are three types of cancers—carcinomas, sarcomas, and the more generalized forms such as leukemias, lymphomas, and myelomas. Carcinomas are the most common. They originate in the epithelial cells that cover tissues, in glandular organs like the breast, and in the mucous membranes that line the mouth, stomach, and lungs. Sarcomas, often highly malignant and consisting of substances like embryogenic connective tissue, are fortunately less frequent. They reside in connective tissue, muscle, bone, and cartilage. Leukemias, lymphomas, and myelomas, rarer still, overproduce respectively white blood cells, lymphoid cells, and bone marrow cells.

How does cancer finally do you in? What is so fatal about it? Several things. A tumor can invade a vital organ like the brain or liver and knock out its life-supporting functions; it may cause a massive hemorrhage by eating through a major blood vessel; a blockage of the kidneys may lead to uremic poisoning; if the stomach is obstructed starvation follows, since parenteral feeding cannot be sustained indefinitely; when a tumor replaces normal lung tissue, the lungs can't get enough air; severe anemia may develop; the unpleasant possibilities are endless. And then the screaming pain if the tumor presses on a bundle of nerves or closes an internal pathway such as the intestines. Sometimes pain is minimal. Yet there's always the terror or impotence as your own body commits suicide against your wishes.

The strain of advanced cancer is so severe that a third to a half of the patients die of infections before the malignancy can finish them off.

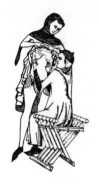

CHAPTER FIVE

The Dilemma
of Breast Cancer

Breast cancer is an exceedingly worrisome disease for women. The female mammary breeds more malignancy than any other anatomical site in either sex. (Lungs in men come in second in overall incidence according to sex.)* One out of seven American women between the ages of thirty-five and seventy

---

*Although the female breast leads in incidence (28 percent versus 21 percent for the male lung), the male lung leads in deaths (31 percent versus 20 percent for the female breast).

will have breast cancer. An estimated 88,000 new cases will be diagnosed in 1975, and approximately 33,000 women will die this year from breast cancer. At current survival rates, which have hardly improved in the past thirty-five years, only 62 percent of breast cancer victims will be alive five years after diagnosis; only 50 percent after ten years.

Why this high mortality? The breast is hardly a vital organ and can be easily spared. Unfortunately, breast tumors tend to go undetected too long. The fatty nature of the site, the instinctive embarrassment of women regarding examinations and unskilled diagnoses by nonspecialists retard early discovery. Pinpoint malignancies can even elude the most expert touch and fool the most perceptive X-ray. So metastasis has a head start in breast cancer. By the time the tumor is noticed, the malignancy has already spread to regional lymph nodes and adjacent tissue in four out of ten cases. However, if the tumor is still localized, the five-year survival rate jumps to 84 percent and declines to merely 73 percent after ten years.

According to a special Gallup poll commissioned by the American Cancer Society in 1973, less than 20 percent of American women regularly do self-examination of their breasts and only half have annual examinations by their physicians. Despite this haphazard pattern, it is the woman who usually detects the lump first.

Some women are more likely than others to contract the disease. They are women who are (1) over thirty-five; (2) have never borne a child; or (3) bore their first after twenty-five; (4) have mothers or sisters with breast cancer; and (5) experienced early menarche and/or late menopause.

The trouble of diagnosis is followed quickly by the trauma of treatment. Surgery is the main recourse for breast cancer. Every woman knows that. But what kind of surgery? Should the whole breast go or just part? You would think doctors would have settled on the most appropriate operation by now, yet they have not. For better or for worse, how much of the breast should be sacrificed is subject not only to medical debate (and surgical advances) but to the sanctions of emotion and even of fashion.

A recent *Vogue* cover (February, 1973) promised to instruct its concerned readers on "How You Can Avoid Breast Surgery." If the hidden assumption here is that a woman could take such advice and live to tell about it, then *Vogue* had one of the medical scoops of the century. In the 1800s, to be sure, the average physician considered breast cancer incurable and recommended against surgery. Shortly before his death in 1892, Dr. Hayes Agnew of the Philadelphia Hospital confessed that he operated on breast cancers solely for the moral effect on his patients. And little wonder. The survival statistics were outrageous. Initial diagnosis usually involved tumors the size of oranges where systemic metastasis was the rule. Even the most pioneering surgeons employing the most advanced procedures of the day could not avoid local recurrences of 60 to 85 percent in their best cases. It was not until Professor William S. Halsted of the Hopkins School of Medicine invented the classical radical mastectomy that recurrence rates began to fall. He simply went farther and deeper with his scalpel in order to "give the disease a sufficiently wide berth." While the German masters Christian Billroth and Richard von Volkmann achieved comparatively good results by resecting the breast, lymph nodes in the armpit, and occasionally the major pectoral muscle, the "Halsted mastectomy" insisted on a painstaking fifteen-step procedure that gutted the chest cavity down to the ribs. The major and minor pectoral muscle, which Halsted deemed expendable, had to go in each case because this allowed for removing all suspected tissue in one neat package. The customary piecemeal dissection seemed to him to increase the chances of leaving a few crumbs of cancer behind. Halsted had to be doing something right because his local recurrence rate—based on fifty operations between 1889 and 1894—dropped to 6 percent. In 1907, he reported the rather astounding news that he was getting a five-year salvage in one out of four breast cancers. Succeeding generations of surgeons slavishly imitated Halsted's technique. With assists from earlier diagnosis and general medical progress, the radical mastectomy achieved 50 percent five-year survival by the 1950s. Some of its better practitioners like Dr. Jerome Urban, acting chief of the breast section at New York's Memorial Sloan-

Kettering Hospital as well as Happy Rockefeller's surgeon, now claim astronomical figures in the nine-tieth percentile for selected series.

Despite the splendid history of the radical, revisionary surgeons have for a long time suggested scrapping it altogether. Halsted needed a "wide berth" for his orange-sized tumors, but such monstrosities would be considered inoperable today when the analogous fruits are more the grape and the prune. The smaller the tumor, the argument goes, the smaller the excision. Just how small in both instances is what the rising smoke is all about. Basically, women have four operations to choose from with or without follow-up radiation: (1) the *radical mastectomy* already described; (2) the *modified radical,* which removes the breast and the nodes but leaves the pectoral muscles; (3) the *simple mastectomy,* which takes the breast alone; (4) the *partial (segmental) mastectomy,* or so-called lumpectomy which merely seeks out the tumor mass and adjacent tissue, although it may carry off up to two-thirds of the breast. But no matter the extent, hardly anybody, including *Vogue* disagrees with Halsted's 1894 dictum that "cancer of the breast is a curable disease if operated on properly and in time."

The *Vogue* story was a breezy apologia by one pseudonymous Rosamond Campion for her struggle to maintain the integrity of her God-given bosom. "Delicately boned, small, lovable, pretty, with a step combining that of Colonel Klink in *Hogan's Heroes* and a Thompson gazelle, she has nothing bizarre about her, except that she shaped her experience in dread illness into something of value for everyone," the introduction hyped. Actually, the *Vogue* item is once removed from Campion's *The Invisible Worm*, a book that has caused more cleavage in breast cancer than anything disputatious surgeons ever wrote up. For Campion assumes the pose of Lincoln Steffens in the slaughterhouse without a firm grasp of the facts. As fiction editor of *Seventeen* (under a second alias, Babette Rosamond) and author of three novels, she was unable to stifle her condemnation of the cancer establishment.

Reduced to its bare bones, *The Invisible Worm* is less the saga of a woman who saved her breast against the odds than the horror in store for females who fail to do likewise. Campion's ordeal started the night she noticed a tiny lump on the inside of her left breast. A cautious sort who had physical checkups twice a year, she went straight to her doctor's office. Indeed the lump seemed suspicious and so she was referred to a breast surgeon. He said the thing was probably benign—nine out of ten lumps are—but that surgery was the only way to make certain. "We'll do a biopsy and we'll know right then and there if it isn't—in which case, of course, we'll go ahead with a radical mastectomy while you're under the anesthetic." The surgeon's nonchalance startled Campion. Two of her best friends had radicals and were never the same again. One cries spontaneously in the middle of otherwise pleasant conversations, the other is in constant pain. A letter from the latter was the ultimate dissuasion: "The nerves in the stump of pectoral muscle are screaming, the burned area gets hot and itchy after the X-ray treatment and develops a thick reptilian hide that sheds grayish-purple flakes for a year. They tell me that cramps and vomiting are psychological. Maybe. All I know is, I was supposed to have a 'topflight' surgeon and a 'topflight' radiologist. Now nearly four years after the operation, I still have an immensely swollen right arm and a chest that sheds gray flakes."

Campion submitted to the knife for her biopsy but wouldn't sign the conventional hospital form permitting the surgeon to go ahead with a radical mastectomy if the growth turned up malignant. Her breast returned from the simple operation intact except for an expendable eight millimeter (one-third inch) tumor and some surrounding tissue. The biopsy revealed malignancy. Undaunted, Campion flew out to the Lourdes of lumpectomies, the Cleveland Clinic, where Dr. George Crile had been preaching the marvels of conservative breast surgery to the consternation of a lot of his fellows. "I'd like every breast cancer patient to be told," Campion quotes him "that there have been random studies made showing that the survival rate after simple mastectomy and radiation is exactly the same as after radical surgery and radiation. And what's more, why not go into it the whole way? Tell these patients that local excision of

early breast cancer yields the same results!" Dr.
Crile opened Campion's breast, found nothing scary,
stitched her back up and sent her home to New York
without a care in the world about her surgical course.

Three years had elapsed since the lady stuck to her
guns and she still wasn't worried when I spoke to her.
Apparently the longer she goes without recurrence,
the cockier she becomes. They all laughed when she
said no to radical mastectomy, but she's getting, it is
hoped, the last laugh now.

If Campion is living proof of the obsolescence of
the radical, why do surgeons continue to perform it?
She gladly informs me in her comfortably elegant
midtown Manhattan apartment—after first lighting up
a cigarette—"They believe in the radical with the
same sincerity that Torquemada believed he could
make people more religious by burning them. The
more they take away from a woman the better they
feel. They might just as well take off your foot
because they don't know where the [cancerous] cell
has gone." She claims that Dr. Crile's lumpectomy
statistics outclass the opposition's. "His survival rate
is much higher than the radicals'." Not so. Dr. Crile
makes a point of saying that his statistics are no
better or no worse than those of surgeons who do
radicals. When I mention the sad fact that most
women who get breast cancer also die of breast cancer despite all known therapies, she balks. "That's not
true. You're quoting NIH [National Institutes of
Health] statistics. Why don't you speak to Crile?"

Then she uncorks an anthropological haymaker in the form of a *New York Times* clipping on an obscure tribe of Ecuadorian centenarians. Healthy as the inhabitants of the valley of Vilcabamba are, they smoke forty to sixty cigarettes a day. "Why do *they* live so long," Campion asks, "when statistics show they shouldn't?"

What irks cancer people about *The Invisible Worm* is the author's egocentric predicament. Although Campion remarked to me that "it would be very cruel and stupid to say that nobody should have a radical and just a local excision," her book allows for the opposite impression. Inquisitorial surgeons bent on mutilation, yellow stuff oozing from her friend's wound, severed breasts in jars outside the Roosevelt Hospital X-ray room—even St. Agnes, the patron saint of breast afflictions, would have second thoughts about the radical mastectomy Campion describes. If you've seen one tumor, you haven't seen them all. Yet nowhere does Campion emphasize the uniqueness of her situation. "Her case is pretty eccentric for two reasons," comments a Memorial Hospital radiologist who specializes in reading breast X-rays. "First, most breast cancer is on the upper outer quadrant because that's where most of the glandular tissue is, but her cancer was on the upper inner quadrant. Second, the size—we don't usually feel tumors that are less than one centimeter. [Campion's tumor measured 8 millimeters, that is, 20 percent smaller than one centimeter.] In one case you can get away with it, but think of all the women who are risking their lives by listening to her."

Why wasn't Campion more scientific in *The Invisible Worm*? "It would have been presumptuous for me to write as a doctor," she replies. "I'm a rather good writer and I was looking for an emotional response in women. The only way to reach people is to appeal to them emotionally and that's what my book has done. I only know me, I can only write about me."

Setting aside the bad faith Campion imputes to sadistic surgeons and bemused statisticians, let's take a look at the operation she dodged.

Andrea Reber* a sixty-year-old Queens housewife, watched Mrs. Campion and Dr. Urban debate the merits of radical breast surgery on the *Today* show. Mrs. Reber reacted immediately by examining her breasts. Ten days later she is lying half-naked in an operating room on the twelfth floor of Memorial Sloan-Kettering Hospital with a tumor of slightly less than two-centimeters in the upper outer quadrant in her left breast. She has given permission for a radical mastectomy, but Dr. Urban guesses a modified will suffice since her axillary nodes appear normal. However, he won't know which it will be until a pathologist puts some of her nodal tissue under a microscope during the operation. At this point even the nature of Mrs. Reber's tumor is in doubt. Neither palpation nor

*The name is pseudonymous.

X-ray is an absolutely safe cancer detector. No surgeon will lop off a breast without a pathologist's say-so. The first step in any mastectomy, then, is to go in and get a chunk of the would-be malignancy.

At 10:55 A.M., Dr. Urban begins the operation by grabbing hold of Mrs. Reber's breast with his left hand and inserting a long, wide needle into the hard tumor with his right. The needle aspirates a tiny portion of tumor tissue, which Dr. Urban scrapes onto a slide. He places the slide in a plastic box and a nurse sends it over to pathology through a pneumatic tube in the corridor. Aspiration saves time—when it works. But the tissue extracted by this method rarely provides conclusive evidence one way or the other and the surgeon will usually have to do a local excision of the whole tumor to satisfy the pathologist.

While Dr. Urban waits for the decision on the left breast, he goes to work on the right. Although Mrs. Reber's right breast appears perfectly normal, he wants to be certain. For women with a tumor in one breast run a high risk of occurrence in the other. Better to catch it now than later. Many surgeons ignore the uninvolved breast on the operating table; others might aspirate it in the general area where the tumor is located on the other side. But Dr. Urban, leaving nothing to fortune, prescribes a full-fledged local excision of 20 to 25 percent of the glandular tissue in the second breast. Since he picks up another cancer in one out of ten patients thereby, he feels the extra surgery is worth the effort. (It is this technique that turned up Happy Rockefeller's pinpoint tumors in the other breast.) The senior of two assisting residents actually does the cutting here. An oval-shaped chunk of yellow-white glandular tissue about three inches long and one inch thick is removed and dispatched to pathology. This precautionary measure does not deform as long as all the surface fat is retained.

At 11:23, the pathologist reports over the loudspeaker that the aspirated sample from the left breast wasn't sufficient to determine malignancy. A local excision will be necessary. The whole tumor Dr. Urban then resects has a dense, fibrous consistency, which, when sliced down the middle, reveals the telltale stellate design of invasive cancer. This specimen follows the same tube route. Word comes back from pathology at 11:34 that the tissue from the right breast is benign. There will be no double mastectomy for Mrs. Reber.

Regrettably, pathologists are human. They don't have the power to see through the microscope's once-in-a-million lie. A renowned breast surgeon confessed an unforgettable whopper to me. A professor's wife came to him with a huge breast tumor. When he opened her he found bad nodes all the way up the axilla. The pathologist's verdict was cancer and a radical mastectomy ensued. After double-checking the specimen in paraffin the next day, the pathologist reversed his decision. The cancer was really tubercular granuloma. Even though the woman lost her breast needlessly, she was so happy it wasn't cancer that she didn't sue. Dr. Urban is prepared for less happier eventualities. He carries $2 million in malpractice insurance—at a yearly premium of $5,000.

"The lesion on left breast is carcinoma," says the pathologist at 11:41. Mrs. Reber is redraped with a sterile gray sheet and the veteran surgeon washes up for his two-thousandth or so mastectomy. Breast surgery may not be unduly complicated, but neither is it to be rushed. Even though no vital organs are endangered or major arteries intersected, the surgeon can't afford to be sloppy with cancer. If he misses only a few microscopic cells, the purpose of the operation could be entirely negated. Consequently, Dr. Urban delicately traces his scapel around the inner contour of Mrs. Reber's flattened left breast, making an elliptical incision above the locale so that the tumor and nipple are in the center of the cut. However, Dr. Urban has to sweep wide to include the nodes in the armpit and those under the pectoral muscles.

It is now 12:20 P.M. This simple procedure has consumed three-quarters of an hour. If pathology pronounces the nodes negative, Mrs. Reber will be sewn up immediately. But if there is a significant degree of cancerous involvement, Dr. Urban will abandon the modified mastectomy and his plan to save the pectoral muscles, and perform the classical radical. Unfortunately the nodes are positive. "Women mind losing their muscles more than their breast," says Dr. Urban, "because they can hide the loss of a breast with a falsie but they can't hide the hollow in the axilla." Dr. Urban goes in to detach the large, meat-red pectoral muscles, the only remaining flesh between Mrs. Reber's skin and ribs. He might have gotten away without the extra surgery. "Most doctors don't do more if they decide on a modified no matter what they find," he remarks, "but I'd hate like hell to think I've left any cancer in there." Dr. Urban quits his chamber at 1:30 P.M. A sadistic procedure? Mrs. Reber, whose life expectancy has just gained several years will have time to decide.

Dr. Urban's smooth Welbian manner packs the customers in. Forty-nine women preceded me into his office early one evening a couple of days after Mrs. Reber's operation, one of a hundred he does each year. The last patient departs at 8:30 P.M. The doctor will sleep right where he is tonight instead of driving home to Scarsdale. A six-figure income soothes the fatigue but six-figure taxes and expenses force him to earn every penny.

So what's it all about between him and his old friend Dr. Crile, emeritus consultant in surgery at the Cleveland Clinic? "The difference between Crile's approach and mine," Dr. Urban comments, "is that I'm really more concerned about leaving disease behind. Honestly, I probably do a little more surgery than I should on the average patient. Take Mrs. Reber's modified radical for example: We found a positive node but we probably won't find anything malignant in the rest of the stuff. I might have quit earlier, but I'd be much happier in my own mind knowing that I've done everything possible to get it all out."

Dr. Urban scoffs at Dr. Crile's contention that conservative surgery is as good as radical. "The trouble with Crile is that he advocates so many goddam different things. . . . He has introduced a sense of chaos into breast treatment. Now any surgeon can do anything he pleases for breast cancer and call upon Crile as his authority. I'm afraid that much of the progress we've made—the 59 percent ten-year salvage at Memorial for all comers with operable cancers and a 98 percent for minimal tumors at five years—will recede if you do all this crappy small stuff."

What American operating rooms need, according to Urban, is a straight law-and-order ticket. "It's a free country, unfortunately," he philosophizes. "Too free. It would be very nice if we had some sort of Academy of Medicine like they do in Russia to set the rules. We don't have enough discipline in the United States. All the stupid people blowing their mouths off and influencing other stupid people—that's why we have all these highjackings and everything else."

If Dr. Urban is behind the surgical times, then Dr. Crile is way ahead. He may be quite right about the obsolescence of the radical mastectomy. If only he could just sustain his objection. Dr. Crile's own cases are hopelessly jumbled and too limited in number to support the unqualified assertion that radical mastectomy is never obligatory. Even one of the surgeons he frequently, though selectively, cites in his own favor, Dr. John Hayward of London's Guy's Hospital, thinks he's frightfully wet. "In spite of twelve years of trial," Dr. Hayward protested during last year's Twelfth Annual Conference on Detection and Treatment of Early Breast Cancer in San Diego, "it is still much too early to recommend local breast surgery instead of radical. As far as I am concerned any surgeon worth his salt will recommend a radical mastectomy."

The consensus seems to be that Crile's intuition and hard sell have outpaced his reasoning. After reading half the manuscript of Crile's *What Women Should Know about the Breast Cancer Controversy,* Dr. Arthur Holleb, the American Cancer Society's vice-president for medical affairs and a retired breast surgeon, dashed off a capsule in-house review: "Sweeping conclusions are not based on sound evidence, too many half-truths and cop-outs when the data show that his approach might be wrong."

A few years ago, Dr. Crile invited NCI statistician Dr. Sidney Cutler up to the Cleveland Clinic to settle his claim once and for all. An independent witness would finally vindicate the superiority of his conservatism. Contrary to expectation, Dr. Cutler came to no conclusion whatsoever. Both the extent and technique of Crile's operations shifted too much from patient to patient and from year to year to pin anything down. "Crile's not running an experiment," Dr. Cutler comments, "but he's trying to draw conclusions as if he were. He's not dishonest. He's just not being logical in a scientific sense." Therefore women ought to beware of illogical and unscientific doctors and their author-patients—the breast you save may haunt you.

Physicians have long realized that the medical miasma surrounding the diagnosis and treatment of breast cancer must be eliminated. The National Cancer Institute is finally doing something to settle the unanswered questions. The same week that Betty Ford was recuperating from her radical mastectomy in Bethesda Naval Hospital last October, breast cancer specialists were gathered across the street at NCI headquarters to report on the preliminary results of various breast management studies.

Dr. William Pomerance of the NCI's Breast Cancer Task Force told the meeting that the first reports on a national effort to document the value of breast examinations—by mammography (a low dose X-ray of the breasts), thermography (a relatively new technique that measures the temperature of the breast for telltale signs of tumor-associated heat), and physicals— indicated that screening may save twenty-two additional lives among every hundred women who have the disease. This estimate was based on a survey showing that 77 percent of women who had mastectomies following screenings had negative armpit nodes as against 40 to 45 percent with negative nodes who had not been screened. This statistic strongly suggests that screening spots breast cancer earlier.

Dr. Pomerance's study revealed that mammography picked up 92 percent of all the lumps which were later found to be malignant, while palpation or physical examination in the same women had discovered only 57 percent. So far, thermography has not proven to be as potent a supplementary diagnostic tool as X-ray. It did, however, pick up 14 percent of tumors which palpation did not detect, but did not detect any which mammography had missed.

If these results hold up across the country in the twenty-seven demonstration clinics that screen women over age thirty-five, it will place many more women in the no-node-involvement category that has an 85 percent probability of a five-year survival. And if screening becomes a standard practice, the breast cancer survival rate could move up sharply from the dismal 62 percent it has been condemned to since the thirties. Dr. Pomerance's estimate comes from analysis of data on 42,000 of the 270,000 women slated for screening at twenty-seven clinics. Financed by NCI and the American Cancer Society, the year-old program will provide free physical, mammographic and thermographic breast examinations for 10,000 women at each clinic, with follow-up examinations in ensuing years.

Results so far prove what clinicians have long suspected—that communities vary in their use of periodic breast exams, in availability of mammographic equipment and X-ray interpreters, and in the aggressiveness with which biopsies are recommended.

The cost of screening is estimated by the ACS at $5,000 per cancer found. "We hope," says Cancer

Society Executive Vice President Arthur Holleb, "that breast screening will become as much a part of good practice as the Pap smear. Deaths from cervical cancer have fallen 60 percent in twenty-five years—much of it due to early detection. If we could achieve a similar reduction in breast cancer, the Number 1 killer of women, that would be good. And if it costs $5,000 to find breast cancer at a curable stage in my wife, it's worth it."

Dr. Pomerance puts the case succinctly: "We hope women will demand periodic screening, the profession will provide it, and the third parties will pay for it."

In another report, the NCI's National Surgical Adjuvant Breast Project (NSABP) compared three different surgical advances to Stage 1 breast cancer (that is, cancer restricted to the breast with no nodal involvement) and learned that radical mastectomy provided no greater protection than less extensive surgery. The standard radical operation, (the one Betty Ford underwent), may be no more effective than less disfiguring surgery in patients where disease did not spread to surrounding nodes.

The NCI-supported nationwide study covering 1,700 patients so far gathers its data from surgeons, radiotherapists, and pathologists at thirty-four clinical centers. The operations being compared are the traditional radical mastectomy, the simple mastectomy, and simple mastectomy plus postoperative radiation therapy.

Dr. Bernard Fisher, the University of Pittsburgh

surgeon who heads the NSABP, stressed that the findings on the major breast operations were still tentative—representing only the first two and a half years of study. So far, all three procedures appear equally effective. Fisher's group declared that less-than-radical surgery is acceptable treatment for primary breast cancer. It is not known yet if the preliminary data will be borne out by long-term follow-up. Many physicians, including Dr. Urban, are still skeptical. After five years the difference in survival rate between radical surgery and conservative surgery may turn out to be negligible. But the ten-year survivals, Urban predicts, will indicate the superiority of the radical. In the meantime, many women will be encouraged to seek the lesser of two evils and could wind up dead for their brave gamble.

Another part of the study compared simple mastectomy plus chest irradiation with standard radical mastectomy for patients with breast and underarm lymph node involvement. The removal of breast tissue followed by postoperative radiotherapy proved just as effective as radical mastectomy.

A critical factor in a breast cancer patient's survival prospects is the condition of her lymph nodes. More than half of all breast cancer patients die with metastatic disease. So removal of the nodes is crucial in getting an accurate assessment of the cancer's extent. If four or more nodes are diseased, the victim's chances of suffering a recurrence within ten years are two or three times as great. Thus the presence of axillary (underarm) gland involvement predicts the presence of metastatic disease. Betty Ford's physicians found cancer cells in two of the thirty lymph nodes removed along with her right breast and pectoral muscles. According to current national statistics, with one to three positive nodes an average 62 percent survival after five years is expected, and after ten years, 38 percent. If four or more nodes are positive, survival is an average 32 percent at five years, and 13 percent at ten years. With no involved nodes, the ten-year survival is 90 percent. Happy Rockefeller's encouraging prognosis owes to the fact that her nodes were disease free.

At the moment, surgery or irradiation or a combination of both are the first weapons a physician uses to attack the primary localized disease. As far as radiation therapy for breast cancer is concerned, Dr. Fisher reports, "There is no evidence anywhere that postoperative radiation therapy improves patient survival following a radical mastectomy." Accordingly, he does not recommend it for Betty Ford. However, Mrs. Ford is taking a mild anti-cancer drug (L-PAM) since two of her nodes indicated the disease had spread.

When cancer recurs, the doctor resorts to such systemic treatment as chemotherapy or hormonal manipulation. Dr. Paul Carbone, chairman of NCI's Breast Cancer Task Force, believes physicians should continue to attack far-advanced disease aggressively with proven combinations of chemotherapeutic agents, along with immunotherapy and hormone therapy. These adjuvants can help improve the quality and duration of life for very ill patients. But, he added, many of these treatments should be used earlier in the course of the disease when better results can be hoped for.

Further clinical studies will be started to evaluate the less extensive surgery known as segmental or partial mastectomy (lumpectomy). The NSABP feels that many women are given partial mastectomies each year although the efficacy of the procedure has not yet been determined. The American Cancer Society notes that lumpectomy isn't necessarily inferior to total surgery. They just say it is unproven. And the ACS presently recommends radical surgery for most cases of breast cancer—and refused to endorse surgery less than removal of the entire breast.

Dr. Crile in Cleveland hasn't done a radical in ten years. The modified radical is still his most common procedure. And now with earlier diagnosis, he thinks the percentage of partials will increase. NCI Director Dr. Rauscher agrees: "I would estimate that well over half of those undergoing breast cancer surgery would be candidates for the less radical procedure."

Hormonal therapy as a postsurgical treatment is given to increase the odds of full recovery. Such therapy may include removal of ovaries, adrenal glands or pituitary glands, a practice which sometimes increases a woman's survival chance by changing her hormonal balance. At the NCI meeting, Dr. William McGuire of the University of Texas in San Antonio reported that hormone receptors—proteins in cancer cells that can be found in breast cancer tissues—can indicate whether these hormonal treatments will be successful. The receptors detect estrogens. The woman may or may not be treated with anti-estrogen drugs or removal of the ovaries if she is premenopausal.

Another development described by Dr. Douglas C. Tormey of NCI is the discovery of three chemical "markers" in the patient's blood that reach abnormal levels when hidden cancer is present. A test for these markers—which together seem to detect 97 percent of the cases in which the patient is still harboring cancer cells—could be used to determine which patients require postoperative therapy and which do not.

Clearly, the dilemma of breast cancer is on the way to resolution. But Dr. Halsted thought so too in 1894.

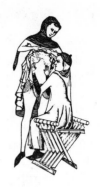

CHAPTER SIX

Lung Cancer

Arthur Godfrey smoked two and one-half to three packs of cigarettes a day for thirty-four years. During the last decade of his smoking, he became deathly ill each morning and could hardly get through his radio show. Godfrey's doctors attributed the nausea to an excess of coffee and orange juice. Following deep hip surgery in 1953, Godfrey discovered he was allergic to the inhalation of smoke of any kind. So he switched to sucking cigars. Unfortunately, sudden abstention does not significantly reduce the risk of

59

lung cancer in heavy smokers who have indulged in twenty years or so of steady smoking (that is, at least a pack a day). It may take thirteen abstinent years to reach the risk level of nonsmokers.

Godfrey's luck ran out in 1959. He felt a gnawing heartburn kind of pain in the area of the heart. A malignant tumor on the upper lobe of his left lung was wrapped around the aorta. Ten years earlier surgeons hardly bothered to operate on lung cancer. (Only 14 percent of lung tumors were considered operable in 1949; 64 percent received no therapy at all.) But since Godfrey appeared free of metastasis, his surgeon resected the upper lobe of his left lung along with the tumor. Six miserable weeks of cobalt treatments and food. "You can't describe the god-awful sickness. You know you're going to die, but you're afraid you won't."

Yet the patient lived. Godfrey belongs to that exclusive fraternity of lung cancer survivors who number only 7 percent after five years and 4 percent after ten. In fact, half of all lung cancer victims are dead within four months following diagnosis. Today, approximately one quarter of all lung tumors are considered operable, another quarter receive no therapy, better than a third get palliative X-rays, and the rest are treated with chemotherapy or combination chemotherapy and X-ray treatments.

Is the cure worse than the disease? Not in Godfrey's case. At seventy-two, he is in excellent shape. The hair is still red and the complexion ruddy. "I can run a little," he says, "I can ride my horse, I can swim, I can scuba, I can fly a plane. I've just slowed down somewhat."

Thoracic surgeon Dr. William G. Cahan is another of Memorial Sloan-Kettering Hospital's radical optimists who won't give a malignancy an even break. Just about any cancer specialist (including the chairman of Memorial's Department of Diagnostic Radiology) will tell you that once the aggressive and hidden lung tumor becomes visible on an X-ray, it's already too late. Dr. Cahan has statistics—on simple and radical lobectomies (removal of one or more lobes respectively) and simple neumonectomies (removal of the lung) and radical pneumonectomies (lung plus lymph nodes)—which prove otherwise. In his hands lung cancer needn't be an immediate sentence of death. "There's a great deal of premature pessimism here. People tend to hang crepe on lung cancer because the overall record is not that good. But by no means should we be defeatists about it. The majority in our survival group have X-rays with shadows on them. If we can get the tumor out, patients have anywhere from a 25 to 60 percent chance for survival. And that doesn't mean everybody dies, does it?" Dr. Cahan insists that his statistics, based on a limited series of 371 operations, are "suggestive but not *compelling.*"

What is compelling about lung cancer is that it is a preventable condition. If only people would stop smoking, the morbid statistics would drop precipitously. Yet despite the blasts of anticigarette propaganda, per capita consumption is on the rise. If this infernal weed were not such a relatively weak carcinogen, the fifty-two million Americans smokers would be in more trouble than they are already. Actually smokers are getting a break they don't deserve. Filter cigarettes are significantly less harmful than the unfiltered brands. Thus the popularity of filtered smoking should be reflected in future mortality statistics.

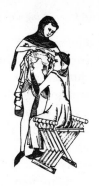

CHAPTER SEVEN

Cancer Modalities: A Treatment Instead of a Treat

When the unmentionable strikes, your options are few and fairly primitive. "Our current means of cancer control are very crude and very physical," comments Dr. Albert Owens, associate physician-in-charge of the Johns Hopkins Hospital Oncology Clinic. "In essence, they amount to—if your right hand offends you, cut it off. And that means you can talk only about parts of the body which you can sacrifice."

Surgery dominates the treatment of solid tumors. Although its marvels are legion, surgery really isn't

63

much better than the cancer sought. A small localized tumor in an accessible site poses little complication. But a larger tumor near or in a vital organ or any malignancy that shows evidence of metastasis has a leg up on any scalpel. Radical surgery can't manage to put a dent in overall cancer mortality rates. Its failure to do so is now forcing surgeons to reexamine the procedures. Why subject a patient to the trial and disfigurement of an extended operation if his survival time is not appreciably lengthened as a result? Some cancer experts go so far as to suggest that the trauma of surgery may shorten life rather than enhance it. In the matter of breast surgery, there is a definite trend toward conservatism. "If the cancer is so advanced that it cannot be removed by an operation less than a radical mastectomy," observes Dr. George Crile in *What Women Should Know about the Breast Cancer Controversy*, "it has already spread through the system and is incurable by surgery." Although the cancer establishment considers Crile an extremist, his alienation from knee jerk operating room radicalism is gradually catching on.

Dr. Edward Reich, an internist turned cancer researcher at Rockefeller University in New York, wishes a pox on all those who perform radical surgery. Breaking protocol with the medical omertà, Reich laces into his colleagues under the skin. "I'm not saying they're crooks, but the only people they're fooling is themselves. The fact is there's no justification for complex therapy. It demoralizes the patient and bankrupts their family." In Reich's view the enemy is the system. "Medicine is ruled by a rigid, wooden, superannuated hierarchy. All these things are decided over lunch at the club. What develops depends on the loudest voice. Science is black and white, so when there's no agreement it's the megaphone. In anything to do with disease, it's almost impossible to get good science because medicine is organized in an unscientific way. They won't let you set up a study to discover what the best treatment is. You can't substantiate radical treatment in breast surgery because the surgeons just yap away. They are, by and large, so arrogant a group that they use people as guinea pigs."

For example, Reich points to a pair of California surgeons whose experimental operations on the bowels of one thousand of the obese led to disastrous consequences. He wouldn't put breast surgeons smack in this category, but he still maintains they are operating without scientific constraints. Improved survival rates don't impress him in the least. "You can't chalk that up to radical surgery, but to diagnosis. We tend to ignore all the advancements in supportive care. People don't realize that all these things help the statistics."

Reich recalls the example of a famous gentleman he knows who has been living with cancer of the lung for twelve years. On the basis of the best medical advice the man elected a small segmental resection of his tumor over the removal of the entire lung. He also refused radiation and drugs. "Lung cancer is supposed to kill you fast," Reich explains, "but radical surgery will kill you faster because it knocks down your immunity. It's when you add on the stress of radical surgery, radiation, and drugs that you hurt the body's resistance to disease."

Tell that to Arthur Godfrey and John Wayne, who are alive and kicking long after waving goodbye to cancerous lungs. "But they're making it at the loss of a lot of other people," Reich replies. "For every instance like Godfrey's and Wayne's, there are people who die in six months instead of three years. And I'm not willing to trade off your three years for Godfrey's twenty. That's stealing a piece of someone else's life. You don't cripple someone with radical surgery with the ephemeral hope of picking up the odd Arthur Godfrey."

While the radical versus conservative debate rages on, both sides would agree with the prophetic declaration of a nineteenth century doctor who said: I do not despair of carcinoma being cured somewhere in the future, but this blessed achievement will, I believe, never be wrought by the knife of a surgeon."

After surgery, radiation therapy is the most common form of cancer treatment. It is generally preferred in skin and head and neck tumors since it can do the job without noticeable damage. Radiotherapy has rescued many tongues and larynxes from unnecessary surgery and subsequent loss of speech. A radiotherapist can reach dispersed cancers like Hodgkin's disease and other lymphomas where the surgeon is helpless. He also mops up postoperatively, seeking out the microscopic leftovers of malignancy. Palliation, however, is radiotherapy's main service. By reducing the size and slowing the spread of tumors, it eases the descent into death.

The X-rays and atomic particles of irradiation are double-edged. The havoc they induce in the chromosomes of cancer cells can also be induced in normal cells. Thus the radiation therapist has to know what he's doing and his machine must be in perfect order. Yet there is a critical shortage in both manpower and equipment. "If all radiation therapy were administered by highly trained full time radiation therapists," one national cancer study notes, "it is estimated that four times the number available would be needed." Given the shortage of trained therapeutic radiologists, the radiation upgrading depends heavily on "outreach" efforts by university radiation therapy centers. For example, the M.D. Anderson Hospital and Tumor Institute has provided radiation physics, engineering, and clinical consultation for six community hospital radiation therapy centers in Texas.

A radiation physicist at the University of Pennsylvania Hospital describes the present circumstances in the United States: "The guy that's doing radiation as a sideline isn't adequate to the task. He hasn't seen enough cancers to know the optimal treatment and optimal equipment is very sophisticated. It can cost up to $200,000, which is beyond the range of most therapists. Expertise is utterly important. The aim is tricky, and to calculate the dosage precisely you need computer planning. We think if you are 10 percent above the optimum dosage you're hurting the patient and at 10 percent below you're not sterilizing the tumor. So without the backup and technical assistance you get at a big center, the little guy can't hack it. You can treat tumors like a schlock or you can treat them as if you know what you're doing. And there are a certain amount of schlocks out there in radiation therapy."

In the fifties and sixties chemotherapy or drug therapy became the rage. A few drugs were actually producing remissions and even bona fide cures in a few bad-acting disseminated tumors. Chemicals were winning where surgery and irradiation could not or feared to tread. Perhaps this was the final breakthrough. If chemotherapy were sufficient to destroy some types of cancer cells, could universal counteraction be far behind? There was no place to go but up and chemotherapists were promising the heights. Someday maybe cancer would be treated by prescription without messy operations or burning rays. Yet two decades later, this hope still remains pie-in-the-sky.

This is not to say, of course, that drugs haven't delivered. On the contrary, in the recent past they are responsible for the most dramatic gains in the treatment of cancer. Choriocarcinoma, a vicious malignancy of the uterus is a perfect instance of both the wonders and limitations of chemotherapy. Before the advent of competent drugs, choriocarcinoma was one of the swiftest and deadliest of all cancers. If a woman had it and didn't get a quick hysterectomy, she was as good as dead in a matter of weeks. Now two drugs by the name of actinomycin D and methotrexate actually offer a *cure* 90 percent of the time; even with distant metastasis to the brain and liver the percentage of cures merely drops to 70. But like every tumor that seems eminently susceptible to chemotheraphy, choriocarcimona is quite rare. In the United States such cases probably do not exceed two hundred a year. Although drugs can assure a normal life expectancy in a majority of patients with several types of fast-growing tumors (Burkitt's lymphoma, childhood leukemia, Hodgkin's disease, etc.), the range of their efficacy is rather narrow. Only fifteen or so cancers (representing less than 5 percent of total incidence in the United States) furnish chemotherapy with a fat target.

Why these kinds and not the others? The explanation is elementary. For maximum kill-power, most drugs have to hit tumor cells while they are in the vulnerable position of division. The more cells divide, the easier they fall. In certain leukemias and lymphomas, a high fraction of the cells is always in some phase of division and thus defenseless. Owing to their slow division rate, however, the major malignancies— lung, breast, colon-rectum, stomach—are impervious to drugs, and treating them chemically is rather iffy. Actinomycin D and methotrexate, like all cancer drugs, have the added attraction of toxicity. Just as irradiation cannot distinguish between normal and malignant cells, neither can chemotherapy. Side effects are as miserable as they are inevitable. Besides saving your life, two three-to-five weeks' actinomycin treatments may also leave you with inflammation and ulcers of the mouth, diarrhea, baldness, mental depression, and bone marrow depression.

Many physicians think—with treatment like this who needs the disease? "It's very common to find patients with tumors we consider curable or at least highly treatable," complains chemotherapist Dr. Vincent DeVita, chief of the National Cancer Institute's Medicine Branch, "who don't receive drugs because they're feeling well and their doctors are unwilling to put them through the rigors of drug therapy at this time—when in fact this may be the only time they have a chance." Dr. DeVita winces as he describes a case he consulted on, a thirty-two-year-old man with carcinoma of the testis. Dr. DeVita recommended immediate chemotherapy, but the doctor in charge hesitated, since his patient seemed in excellent health. Six months later DeVita was called in again. The tumor had metastasized to the lung. "He gets his lung resected," DeVita says, "and six months later there's evidence of metastasis in the other lung. But he's still feeling fine. What do you do? There are three or four drugs for this, but the cure rate is 10 percent. The odds are nine to one you'll fail." So chemotherapy was again rejected, this time on the grounds that the patient was a goner anyway so let him go in peace. "This wasn't done from maliciousness," DeVita explains in exasperation. "They were just trying to protect him from those awful drugs. But where the hell was his therapy? That guy didn't have a chance."

Notwithstanding the checkered history of chemotherapy, drug research commands special priority at the National Cancer Institute. NCI is where it all began in the mid-fifties when pharmaceutical houses decided the r&d of cancer drugs wouldn't pay its way in profits. The tycoons were right. At a staggering cost, NCI has turned up only forty-two cancer-fighting drugs in nineteen years. In 1972, for example, NCI spent $75 million testing 30,800 natural and synthetic chemicals as potential anticancer agents. Of these several thousand compounds, just four were accepted for human experimentation.

Twenty million dollars is a far-out price for one drug, but NCI has its back against the wall. "Surgery and radiation have reached a dead end," insists Dr. Gordon Zubrod, NCI's pioneering chemotherapist and director of its Division of Cancer Treatment. "As more and more drugs became effective, there emerged the notion that the best method for treating cancer is to use everything you have and that the best clues for reducing mortality is surgery plus chemotherapy or surgery plus irradiation." Combination therapy, then, is the official wave of the future.

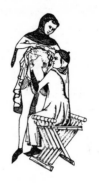

CHAPTER EIGHT

Immunotherapy: The Last Promise?

Why isn't cancer more ubiquitous? If it's nasty enough to shake down one out of four, why not four out of four? Or does it happen that some of us are cancer prone and others cancer resistant? It certainly does. The kicker appears to be the body's immune system, nature's way of telling foreign substances to bug off. Without this biological DEW line we would be mincemeat for millions of infectious micro-organisms. The immunological surveillance system runs on lymphocytes, the white corpuscles manufactured in the bone marrow and stored in the lymph glands and nodes. Lymphocytes come in two models: B-cells synthesize free-circulating antibodies to do battle with bacterial invaders while T-cells concentrate on larger insults like transplanted tissue and organs. Once the lymphocytes notice something odd, they rush to the trouble spot and do their duty. Occasionally macrophages or scavenger cells lend an assist by cannibalizing the trespasser.

How does cancer collide with the immune system? Tumor cells can usually be recognized as alien. Besides all the other things that make them malignant, tumor cells display unique surface proteins (antigens) that the host regards as nonself. As long as the lymphocytes stay on top, the theory goes, cancer will be kept in Sisyphean check. But if immunological surveillance is impaired, incipient malignancy may go over the top. "In order for cancer to occur and persist there must be a failure of the immunological process," states immunologist Dr. Robert Alan Good, president and director of the Memorial Sloan-Kettering Cancer Center. "We've never found a cancer patient in whom something wasn't screwed up immunologically."

Clinicians have only recently begun to exploit the programmed aggression of the immune system against cancer. A therapeutic agent like BCG has an immunologic rationale—to challenge the body's defense mechanism with alien microorganisms in the hope that the local immune response will destroy the neoplasm. Dr. Edmund Klein of Roswell Park Memorial Institute in Buffalo tripped over the possibility in one of those happy accidents of medical discovery. As a young doctor, Klein did research on leukemia with the late Dr. Sidney Farber of Boston's Children's Cancer Research Foundation. But leukemia was a tough nut and Klein felt stymied. "It's hard to learn what goes on when you're working with the critical stages of the disease," he says. "At that point you're throwing in everything. I preferred to look at a simpler cancer—skin cancer—which is accessible and relatively benign. At worst, if you make a mistake, you can go back and correct it. There is enormous flexibility."

In 1960, Dr. Klein was giving large amounts of drugs to his patients orally, hoping that some of the chemicals would reach the skin. Then he decided to apply the drugs experimentally on the site itself. This variation succeeded in killing the tumors. In the course of the experiment, however, Dr. Klein incidentally observed that some drugs produced allergies on the skin and that the allergic reactions were more intense in the tumor area. After swelling and blistering, the tumors would completely disappear and healthy tissue would regrow in their place. This wasn't the doing of chemotherapy; it was a historic manifestation of the immune system's ability to defeat cancer. So far, two hundred cutaneous cancer patients have been treated with immunotherapy at Roswell Park (where Dr. Klein moved in 1961). Five-year studies of Dr. Klein's original twenty-four patients indicate that 95 percent of their cumulative five thousand skin lesions went into total remission.

Attempts to extend immunotherapy to other cancers have not borne out. Even so, the anecdotal data augurs reasonably well. Dr. Klein had five cases of previously untreatable breast metastasis in partial regression through immunotherapy when I spoke to him in early 1973.

BCG is being tried in cases of acute leukemia of childhood and malignant melanomas. Further studies, however, are needed to establish the effectiveness of this approach. Immunotherapy with BCG scored its first successes with the leukemias as pioneered in the BCG trials of Dr. George Mathé in France, and recently confirmed by the Medical Research Council of Britain. BCG, a nonspecific immune response stimulant, is now undergoing trials with solid tumors, notably melanomas. Other facets of the immune system are also being studied for possible clinical effect. But they are largely limited to patients with advanced disease for whom other modalities have failed.

Across the board, however, the betting is still rather light. Dr. Klein candidly outlines the shortcomings of our immune system in the following manner. "First, it's terribly complex; second, it's liable to go wrong in several ways: (a) we can lose its presence through viral disease; (b) the antigenic difference between normal and abnormal cells may be so subtle that the system doesn't see the latter as foreign; (c) it may just be a crummy system in the sense that the antibodies we develop sometimes protect the tumor instead of fighting it; and (d) being a real monster, cancer has the means of inhibiting the activity of cells that would destroy it. When you speak of immunologic impairment, you're speaking of a range of qualitative and quantitative defects."

Immunotherapists are undaunted. For example, Dr. Jordan U. Gutterman of the M.D. Anderson Hospital and Tumor Institute in Houston, compares the present fledgling state of immunotherapy with that of chemotherapy in the late forties, and he expects the newcomer to catch up with its predecessor as a cancer treatment within the next five years.

NCI's chemotherapist-in-chief Gordon Zubrod disagrees. "Immunotherapy has yet to cure the first patient," he points out. "When and if they show some of the experimental work in animals carries over to man, then the comparison may be true. I'm sure they don't mean that immunotherapy should be in widespread use for man, since it can enhance tumor growth."

Dr. Klein's labors don't exactly knock Dr. Zubrod off his chair. "There are a few cases in which he's seen dramatic results," concedes Dr. Zubrod, "but none in which we've seen the life history of tumors. These isolated cases don't prove that immunotherapy is a good primary form of cancer therapy. There are certain theoretical and factual difficulties that make me personally doubt it's going to be as happy a way of treating cancer as its enthusiasts make out. For instance, the killing power of immunotherapy is never enough to make the tumor disappear. You're dealing with trillions of cells in human cancer. Therefore, it looks as though immunotherapy will have to be used with something else."

Dr. Klein, of course, will not yield. "The way to change an anecdote into a phenomenon is with money," he retorts. "And money we haven't got. We get some support from NCI, but not enough. Every evidence we have indicates that immunotherapy works on a spectrum of cancers, and the extent to which it works depends on how much we look. We haven't even scratched the surface." Another immunotherapist remarks irately, "If Gordon Zubrod has the data to show the shortcomings of immunotherapy, he ought to publish it. But if all he has is a hunch, then he ought to shut his mouth."

As low man on the totem pole of cancer treatment, immunotherapy is prey to professional prejudice. More serious, however, is the moral hurdle. In animal models immunotherapy can lay waste a tumor when it's so big, but fails when the tumor is just a fraction bigger. Thus the optimum circumstance for using immunotherapy is after the mass of the tumor has been reduced by some other therapy or—here comes the dilemma—while the mass is still very small. "When a tumor is on the way up," comments Dr. William D. Terry, head of NCI's immunology branch, "you have a little ethical freedom to try experimental approaches when other known therapies can have some effect. The only place where you pick up your possibilities is with people who are going to die anyway."

In the final analysis and despite the best of intentions, surgery, irradiation, chemotherapy, and immunotherapy aren't yet doing the greatest job keeping body and soul together. When you're rolling against the Big Casino, the odds are still with the house.

So what else is new? Everyone knows that malignancy isn't a bed of roses. At least we can suffer and die with the consolation that American medicine in its infinite wisdom and resources has pulled out all stops in our behalf. This hope is the opiate of the victims. Perhaps it's better for them to believe in the sanctifying grace of their doctors than to be told the depressing truth. "The treatment of cancer in the United States," says a senior member of NCI's hierarchy, "really is deplorable. Advanced cancer is something for the dedicated specialist who is familiar with the advantages of different therapies. We've grown up in a medical monolith in this country. Even in the big centers cancer is looked upon not as what's best for the patient but what's best for my specialty. One reason this happens is because med schools are built on departments and when you get to be chairman you're a big wheel and people jump. You tend to conserve that delightful situation, so much so that you don't feel comfortable when somebody suggests that medicine ought to fit the patient. The monolith has prevented disciplines from cutting across department lines—all interns are trained like the chairman. But the treatment of cancer depends on the cooperation of several disciplines."

The NCI's approach to the treatment of cancer may be taking on some changes since Dr. Alfred S. Ketcham retired as chief surgeon on July 1, 1974. The youthful thirty-three-year-old Dr. Steven A. Rosenberg succeeds him following a five-year internship and residency in surgery at the Peter Bent Brigham Hospital in Boston. Dr. Rosenberg, who spent two years doing research at the NCI immunology branch, sees cancer surgery as playing two continuing roles in the still unknown future of what he calls "innovative therapy." One is its conventional function in excising bulk disease "to every last cell that surgery is capable of removing." The other is to provide the immunotherapists with tumor tissue for use in developing "adjunctive mechanisms to somehow trick the immune response into performing a practical role in cancer therapy." Yet he insists that the "practical answers are more likely to come from the clinical surgeon than a research immunologist, because the surgeon is devoting every thought to his patients."

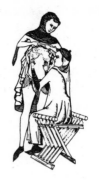

CHAPTER NINE

In Case of Cancer

If you come down with one of cancer's seven warning signals—unusual bleeding, a thickening in the breast or elsewhere, indigestion or difficulty in swallowing, nagging cough or hoarseness, a sore that won't heal, change in bowel or bladder habits or an obvious change in a wart or mole—your life may depend on how fast you can remove yourself to a major cancer facility. Nothing less is advised. Don't rely on your family physician who probably didn't notice the cancer early enough anway. In 1929 the American So-

81

ciety for the Control of Cancer issued a sober warning that still holds today: "We have been forced to conclude that the treatment of many major forms of cancer can no longer be wisely entrusted to the unattached general physician or surgeon or to the general hospital as ordinarily equipped. . . ." The chairman of the President's Cancer Panel, Dr. Benno Schmidt, knows best. "If I had a cancer," Schmidt commented at the 1974 American Cancer Society's annual science writers' seminar in St. Augustine, Florida, "I would get to a medical center that specializes in that kind of cancer."

Where do you drop in for superlative diagnosis and care? Regrettably, your choices are thin. There aren't more than a handful of cancer centers—such as Roswell Park in Buffalo and M.D. Anderson in Houston—that provide the medical maximum. If you can afford the room rate, which can run over $200 a day, you should do what Babe Ruth, Brian Piccolo, Eddy Duchin, Van Johnson and Happy Rockefeller did—you should reserve a bed in Memorial Sloan-Kettering Hospital on Manhattan's Upper East Side. People are literally dying to get in. Patients fly up from South America and arrive unannounced at the hospital's doorstep. Relatives send terminal cases over in ambulances hoping a miracle will be pulled off. The place has a last-resort reputation, an image it would be glad to shuck off, or at least reduce. Memorial's staff is deservedly proud of saving patients who have been condemned to premature death by other doctors in other facilities. But they often have to try harder since they receive so many advanced cancers. Hence the pesthole publicity. Throughout its ninety-year history, the institution has been accustomed to having its surgical approach alternately praised as heroism and criticized as extremism.

Memorial's superiority complex feeds on its crackerjack team of 150 specialists and its utterly sophisticated multi-million-dollar equipment. The average community hospital is a Civil War M.A.S.H. unit in comparison. The botched referrals which filter into Memorial testify to the barber-doctoring that often obtains in cancer treatment. "We not only have all kinds of cancer experts," asserts Memorial's Chief Medical Officer Dr. Edward J. Beattie, Jr., "but we have experts in every field that medicine has experts in who can also take care of cancer." To assure that this abundance of expertise doesn't clash at the patient's expense, the hospital has stamped out competition among specialists by instituting a fixed-salary-plus-expenses arrangement for its full-time attendants. Financially, Memorial staffers are no longer tempted to impose their specialty on their private patients. Their motto is: To each according to scale and from each according to the patient's necessity. "We've developed a triage system here," says Dr. Thomas J. Fahey, Jr., Memorial's director of Outpatient Services, "whereby every patient is evaluated by a surgeon, a radiologist, and a chemotherapist. When they were in private practice and income depended on their own patients their judgment was different. It's a hell of a lot different today. Nobody's got an ax to grind."

Memorial Hospital's tradition for radical surgery—it pioneered the semi-corporectomy, a now discarded operation that left a person with little below the chest—encourages bold experimentation. For example, liver cancer has a five-year relative survival rate of 3 percent and commonly kills in a couple of months' time. Surgery is more effective than drugs but the surgeon can't resect the whole liver. Oh no? Dr. Joseph G. Fortner, chief of Memorial's Transplantation and Gastric and Mixed Tumor Services, believes the day of liver transplants is here. In addition to inventing safe procedures for more radical liver surgery (removing up to 80 percent of the organ), Dr. Fortner is heading a drive to make transplantation respectable as a cancer treatment. In 1969, his team performed six transplants; the longest survival was a disappointing but world-record nine months. Then their grant ran out and was not renewed. "This hospital is very demanding," he said in the winter of 1973. "You're supposed to do something perfect the first time. We were shut down until last fall and now we're laboriously starting up again. And it looks like we've got a home run."

The surgical four-bagger cited was a then four-year-old boy who received a heterotopic, or auxiliary, liver transplant in December, 1972. Four months later the kid was going strong. "I am very hopeful about liver

transplants for cancer patients," remarked the buoy-
ant Dr. Fortner. "There's every reason to expect a
goal like present-day kidney transplants."

Treatment is only as good as the original diagnosis.
At Memorial Hospital your cancer has little chance of
hiding. Dr. Robin Watson, the British-born head of
Memorial's Diagnostic Radiology Department, pre-
sides over an eerie array of X-ray equipment. Not one
of his expensive machines actually treats a patient.
His task is to diagnose, that is, to search for the
tumor that others will later try to destroy. Having
viewed too many mistaken readings of other radiologists, Watson is dismayed with the state of his specialty.

"The accent in this day is upon quantity rather
than quality," Watson told me. "Particularly the field
of cancer detection, it would be better to have a
reasonable number of superbly qualified radiologists
rather than an unlimited number of 'observers.' Such
a state depends upon the ability of the largest centers
where teachers and expertise are concentrated. Unfortunately in recent years, we have reached the position
where as a result of increasing expenses and lack of
support the universities are no longer able to maintain
large teaching services, and in many instances, the
number of radiologists under training has had to be
limited. The burden of training has, therefore, fallen
upon those smaller centers which are less well-
qualified to embark upon the necessary rigorous
training programs. I would judge that at least 30

percent of the X-rays performed are unnecessary in the management of a patient. This wasteful expenditure of energy on the part of the radiologist and money and time on the part of the patient is directly attributable to the power and persuasion of the jurist. It is a sad reflection that the vast majority of X-rays are taken just in case a lawsuit may result. How much better if this energy would be expended in the search of cancer.

"Recently there has been a trend sponsored by the health authorities to recognize only those cardiac centers which can prove their proficiency by virtue of a number of patients treated. There is no place for the occasional, though enthusiastic and possibly well-motivated operator without the backing of an expert team. The same is true to a certain extent of arteriography in the field of radiology. All too often cases have to be repeated on referral because of the inadequacies of the result. This involves the patient again in extra expense and trauma. Better that such cases be referred to large centers where specialists in such fields exist, thereby eliminating the vast expense incurred by smaller centers in the establishment of underutilized suites controlled by inadequately trained individuals."

Perhaps the comparison between Memorial Sloan-Kettering Hospital and all but a handful of other cancer centers will not be so odious in the future. However, unless such Memorial-type facilities increase and multiply, the advances in cancer care will be for almost nothing.

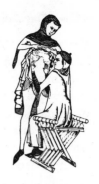

CHAPTER TEN

How Far Do You Go?

For women over forty-five, cancer of the ovaries usually means death. The median survival time for this age group is a little more than a year. So how far do you go to save your mother from dying of ovarian cancer? This question never occured to Frank and Charlotte Friedman. They decided Charlotte's mother would live despite a discouraging prognosis and the inevitable roadblocks medical men reflexively set up when outsiders encroach on their territory.* "Every-

*The names of persons, hospitals, experimental treatments (except alkarin and BCG) and locations in the following story have been

thing we did," they stressed, "was through established medical institutions—none of this stand-on-your-head-twice quackery." Yet some of the finest cancer centers in the United States treated Charlotte Friedman and her mother shamefully. Cancer seems to bring out the best and worst in people. And no wonder.

The Friedmans reside in Cleveland. They are in their mid-thirties and have one child. Their four-room apartment is a hanging garden of lush plants and Picasso and Miro lithographs. Frank makes good money in a small partnership. Charlotte, a delicately beautiful feminist, is presently between careers. I spent five hours with the couple one night hearing their story. The daughter's pain has not yet subsided. Charlotte recalled the six months' nightmare with sudden and extreme shifts of mood—anger, impotence, pity, sadness, rage, and contempt. Frank listened supportively, occasionally correcting a fact or injecting a name. Once or twice when he attempted to take over the narrative, Charlotte shut him up. For her, the telling is therapy.

Mrs. Julie Schwartz, Charlotte's mother, who lived in Detroit, had a hysterectomy at forty-five and a radical mastectomy at forty-nine. Nobody ever informed her she had cancer; they said the breast was "suspicious." Charlotte insists her mother didn't want

changed. The distances between cities and countries, however, are approximately the same, as are all other details.

to know and the charade was maintained by her father and brother, both doctors themselves. Some years after the mastectomy, Mrs. Schwartz developed an inconsequential lip cancer which was remedied by surgery. In 1970, an exploratory operation revealed ovarian cancer. The surgeon closed her up without removing the diseased ovary. Metastasis was too widespread, he said. He gave Mrs. Schwartz a year.

"For two weeks I was berserk," said Charlotte. "Then one day my father telephoned from Detroit and said, 'I solved it.' He had been calling hospitals all over the country about chemotherapy and settled on alkarin, which is a drug they use for ovarian cancer at the Grimm Institute. He didn't want a drug that would make her hair fall out, which was what they wanted to give her at the Detroit Hospital. He said, 'The alkarin should shrink the tumor up and then one year later we reoperate. She's going to make it.'

"A few weeks later I was in Detroit reading through the literature on alkarin. It showed that only 30 percent have a remission on it. My father was being too optimistic. I got so upset after I read that. I thought there must be something else. Then Frank and I, but mostly Frank, went into intensive research on cancer unbeknownst to my father, who insisted on staying with conventional medicine. First, I should say we had to do it on our own. My mother's surgeon, for example, pronounced her dead and never saw her ever again, EVER.

"Well, Frank contacted Dr. Richard Burns, who's the head of research at the Ferrell Cancer Institute in Cleveland. He told us a lot about immunotherapy, which is supposed to build up the body's immune system instead of breaking down the cancer. Burns was working with Navien's toxin and expected a fresh shipment in from France in a couple of months. He said his stuff was absolutely terrific and that my mother could be part of an experimental program blah blah blah.

"Before going on, I have to tell you that with the exception of Richard Burns every doctor we wrote to wouldn't answer us. Each replied with curt letters saying, 'You're not a physician. If you wish to get in touch with us, you must have a physician write.' At that time my father wouldn't help and no other doctor would listen to us. They had already buried her. And the ones who hadn't wouldn't go beyond traditional chemotherapy. In fact, they all laughed at us. I don't remember if we forged names, but when my mother got bad we finally convinced my father. We called a doctor in Portland. We called a doctor in Birmingham.

"Each researcher criticized the other. One would say don't go to *him* because *his* drug is no good. They all led us to believe that theirs was the real thing. These doctors are so competitive, and they don't have anything. They should say, 'God, try anything.' But they don't. So each one runs the other down.

"We probably sent sixty letters and made a hun-

dred phone calls a month. We called and called and
called and called. Then a friend of mine who's a
brilliant physicist remarked to me: 'You're the kind
of person who destroys it for the rest of us. You take
up too much of the researcher's attention. He doesn't
have time to be bothered by people like you. Your
mother's going to die. Let her die.'

"Meanwhile it's April and my mother hadn't gone
into a slide yet. But I thought the minute she does, I
must have something ready immediately or even con-
currently. My father and I were having violent argu-
ments. My father is a wonderful man, but he was
terrified about trying something experimental. Every
day we'd leave the house and I'd say, 'Daddy, try
these drugs, try them.' Because all these doctors make
you feel they have this fantastic thing. And it's always *just* coming in.

"We finally latched onto this doctor in Salt Lake
City. He sounded the most hopeful, but he was just
setting up his institute and needed money for a new
batch of drugs. We asked him how much. He said
$4,000. We said, 'It's yours.' Then something went
wrong. One day he informed us that he would treat
my mother only if she went out to Salt Lake City. We
even invented a rare but curable blood disease to get
her out there because she still didn't know she had
cancer. Then the doctor raised another obstacle—my
mother would have to sign a letter which read: 'I
Julie Schwartz know that I have well-differentiated
ovarian carcinoma and that I am willing to risk my

life. . . .' My father said, 'Go to hell. She'll *never* sign
it.' We pleaded with him to waive the letter. We said,
'Can't you have her sign a copy that doesn't contain
that sentence and then . . .?' No. He didn't care and
that was the end of him.

"And do you know that every doctor remarked
that the ovary should have been removed in the first
place? They said immunotherapy works when it's a
smaller tumor. They just couldn't *believe* the surgeon
at the Detroit Hospital didn't take anything out.
Then we began to hear of case after case of remission
when the tumor was operated on. I begged them to
operate on her again, but they wouldn't.

"The doctors in Detroit never even heard of immunotherapy. I told my brother about it and he said
it was quackery: 'If it's so good, why isn't it in the
papers?' Well, now it's in the papers. They're just
surgeons so they didn't know that if you take out the
ovary there might be a chance with immunotherapy.
In fact, the Salt Lake City doctor wasn't going to
treat her unless she had another operation.

"Next thing—Frank's partner finds a doctor in
Pittsburgh who says he has the rich man's cure for
cancer—a series of injections called L-10 at $250
each. Then I did some reading about BCG. All this
time my mother seems to be improving on alkarin,
but we have Navien's toxin, the rich man's cure, and
BCG ready as backup.

"In May I get a call: Mother feels a pain. The word
is, the end. The tumor was massive and they expected

a bowel closure imminently. I wanted to try all these new treatments. Everyone said to let her die in peace.

"The guy in Pittsburgh, the one with the cure, kept promising the injections for next week, the next week. Finally, he said, 'I have it but I can't give it to you. It's for rats.' Well, Frank screamed so loud, 'This woman is blown up. She may not be alive in six weeks. Goddamit, let us have it.' The guy said okay. So the next day I get on a train for Pittsburgh. Then in his office the doctor explains that he's tried L-10 on animals, but he doesn't know if it's good for humans. The two persons he used it on both died, but he'll see if it works on my mother. Who the hell is this doctor to bring me down there for that? THE TWO PEOPLE HE GAVE IT TO DIED. All along he's been telling us it's a *cure*.

"So I take this vial—L-10 can't be exposed to heat, light, or movement—and I'm fanning it on the hundred-degree train. I switch at Cleveland and get another train to Detroit. My father meets me at the station at eleven at night and races to a drugstore to buy a syringe. My mother's lying in the Detroit Hospital with a big bloated belly and he puts it in. I remember her crying. She then blows up tremendously.

"While this is happening—it's the end of June now—a friend from the Ferrell Cancer Institute shows me an unpublished paper by a Doctor Tretkov from Estonia. I couldn't believe it. In the thirties, Tretkov noticed that Estonians don't get cancer very much and he checks their diet. Then he comes up with the idea that there's some anticancer substance in Estonian yogurt. He isolates it out for twenty years and shows that when he gives the yogurt bacillus to animals there is *complete* cure of cancer in every case. When he gives it to people, you couldn't believe it. He had one case of a guy in a uremic coma with cancer of every bone in his body and he brought him back. Some of his patients were dead, in comas for two weeks ready to crock out, but they recovered with his injections. Ovarian cancer, much worse than my mother's, and he saves them. I start to cry. She's cured.

"For three solid weeks we tried to place a call to this guy. But we couldn't get through. We sent about twenty-two cables.

"Meantime I read that BCG can be effective if it's injected right into the tumor. My brother said, 'Charlotte you're titched. Who ever heard of BCG?' Some immunotherapist gives her BCG on the skin of the abdomen and she develops a pox. Then my father suggested we might be able to get to the tumor if we go up through the vagina. What a cool idea. He asked a friend to do it, but the friend refused. Some place in the world, I told him, there's a doctor who will do this. He said, 'I just can't risk mother's life for this.' And I'm saying, 'Daddy, gamble, gamble, Daddy. What have we got to lose?' He said, 'I can't murder my wife. I can't murder my wife.' He got no support from his colleagues at the Detroit Hospital. They thought he was nuts and that I was some witch.

"Then one Saturday morning after I pleaded un-successfully with the immunotherapist to administer the BCG directly—they'd rather my mother die than try anything unconventional—I made reservations for Estonia and flew out Sunday morning. My father didn't know about it because I knew he'd kill me. I get there"—Charlotte begins to sob lightly—"this really upsets me, it's the worst part . . . and just catch Tretkov because he's leaving for Japan the next day. He shows me his mice and his chart of 347 successful cases. Then he said to me, 'Your mother will be well.'

" 'You mean if . . .' I said.

"He said, 'But she will.'

" 'Then you're telling me you have the cure for cancer.'

" 'Oh, I can't say that but I have great hope. . . .' A very humble man.

" 'But if this is a cure, the world must know. Why haven't you given it out?'

" 'Tomorrow I am going to a pharmaceutical house in Japan and if they get the same results as I am getting, and they will, you will then hear about it all over the world.'

"He gave me packages and packages of this crap in a powder. When I asked him why I couldn't have the serum which is injected into the mice, he said it was too powerful. 'First your mother must take this powder and the tumor will shrink. Then she will come here and I will give her the serum, but if I give it to her now, the cancer cells will release so much poison that she will die.'

"I called Frank from Estonia and said, 'I knew I'd cure her. I knew I'd cure her. I knew I'd cure her.' And I used to tell my father that if she gets everything, something should work because we'd hear about something that worked on somebody and another thing that worked on somebody else. On the plane to New York I stuffed the powder in my bra and underpants in case I couldn't get the cartons through customs. However, there was no trouble. I went right through with the cartons and caught a plane to Detroit.

"Frank met me at the airport and raced the powder to the Detroit Hospital, where my mother was all blown up again. They had to sneak it in because it wasn't FDA-approved. I go running up the following day and say, 'Mother, here's your life in this bag.' And she wept and I wept. Everybody except my father, my mother, Frank, and myself thought we were *absolutely* loony bins.

"Tretkov promised there would be immediate effects, but after two weeks of daily doses she's not getting any better. So Frank cables Tretkov in Japan. Tretkov replies that we should increase the dosage. He says my mother's cells are probably being killed off too fast. Then we tell him we're desperate, desperate for the serum. He replies that he might be able to come to New York and give my mother the serum if he feels it's necessary. We paid his expenses here and pretended it was the Ferrell Cancer Institute. The Institute was interested in seeing him, but they wouldn't pay his way.

"It's now August. My father and brother drive my mother down from Detroit the day Tretkov arrives. He spends the whole day with my father and brother on our terrace diagramming what he's going to do for my mother. He said, 'She's going to make it. Don't listen to America. It doesn't respect life, but life is very important to us in Estonia.' We asked him to take her to Estonia for treatment, but he wouldn't hear of that.

"That night my mother was the worst. She needed to be tapped. Frank brought her into the Ferrell Hospital as an outpatient. They treated her like a dog there. They wouldn't even let Tretkov in her room. They hardly spoke to him."

After two hours of nonstop talking, Charlotte passed to Frank, who stayed with his mother-in-law at Ferrell that day. "Around four o'clock in the afternoon she was so weak she couldn't get up. But Ferrell Hospital didn't want to admit her. She had to have one of their doctors admit her but she didn't have one there. It was procedure. They also would not give her plasminate to replace the fluids lost in the tapping. They said she had forty-eight hours and to get her home. We finally got a doctor to admit her.

"At some point or other I took Tretkov over to see Dr. Richard Burns, the Institute's research director. He presented his Navien's toxin charts. . . ."

"And then," Charlotte interrupted, "Tretkov said something at that meeting he didn't say in Estonia— that he had a chart of 347 failures to go with the 347 successes he showed me. So his yogurt cure wasn't

100 percent effective but only 50 percent effective."

"The discussion went well," Frank resumed. "Tretkov asked the hospital to treat her mother experimentally according to his regimen. They wouldn't do it. They couldn't permit a foreign doctor in the hospital."

"The clinician on my mother's case," Charlotte interrupted again, "called Tretkov something like a spic. They were so mean at Ferrell. My brother came down from Detroit and they wouldn't even let him look at her chart. He said, 'It's my mother and I'm a physician.' And they said, 'Butt out, buddy. Who the hell do you think you are?' Then my brother asked the clinician if he wouldn't like to look at the chart if it were his mother in another hospital and the guy answered no."

"Mind you," Frank adds, "the Ferrell Cancer Institutes is one of the three best cancer centers in the country and we had to get her out of there for her own good. They wouldn't even give her the proper nutrients intravenously. So we brought her back to Detroit Hospital in an ambulance."

"Meanwhile," Charlotte went on, "Tretkov says, 'So long, guys,' and flies back to Estonia. At Ferrell the doctors said she would die in forty-eight hours, but they gave her the proper replacements in Detroit and she lived for six more weeks.

"Even at Detroit we were administering Tretkov's powder. We still weren't sure it wasn't working. We had to sneak it in and then devise ways to get the nurses out of the room. Sometimes my mother wouldn't take it and we got it into her rectally through enemas. My father went through this incredible strain because the doctors, men my father taught, made him feel like he was from Mars. The nurses yelled at my mother. They cursed her. I tried to get my father to fly my mother to Estonia because Tretkov is constantly cabling that she's going to make it. 'You have to get the poisons out,' he insisted. 'The worse she's getting, the better she's getting.' I still believed in Tretkov. We wanted to keep her alive and they didn't. If my brother wasn't there every day, she would have died five weeks earlier.

"Towards the end, my mother stopped taking it. She got worse and worse. The cancer had eaten through the bowel. My father and I started to pour buckets of the powder down a tube in her throat. We weren't afraid of the poison anymore. She had been getting just bits of it at Detroit because we thought we may have given her too much before. Tretkov didn't know the right dosage. Frank began sending wild cables to Estonia, 'Help, help, we don't know what to do.' And we never heard from Tretkov again, nor did he ever inquire whether she lived.

"At two o'clock on September 22, a nurse named Stempleski, who had befriended my mother, told me to get my father quick. She was in a coma and her pulse was sinking. My mother was gone by three o'clock but she hadn't been pronounced officially dead. Then the next nurse, Miss Jalet, came on duty.

This is the one who told my mother we were crazy. My sister, who arrived earlier, says to her, 'We won't need you today. My mother's dead.' Right after this the head nurse comes in and says, 'Miss Stempleski, leave this room.' Outside in the corridor she told her off. 'Miss Stempleski, how dare you overstay your service? You're fired.' My father is weeping because my mother's dead and the nurses are screaming outside because we had broken all protocol because we didn't switch nurses at three o'clock. I asked the head nurse if she had ever lost a mother. 'Don't give me your emotions,' she screamed. 'You have disgraced the name of Miss Jalet.' That's the last thing I heard at that hospital."

"The most important part of the story," Frank concluded, "is that the autopsy showed that the tumor was just like every other ovarian tumor. Tretkov's yogurt powder hadn't done a damn thing, zero."

"There's something more important that that," Charlotte added. "One year later, BCG and immunotherapy had become the most promising cancer treatment. Injecting into the site of the tumor—which nobody would do—now is about the only thing they do. But nobody ever said they goofed. They just say, 'Your mother never had a chance.' "

"The clinician absolutely hates the experimental researcher and the researcher won't let you know what's going on unless you're a doctor," Frank commented. "I wouldn't have gotten to first base if I hadn't told them I was connected with a foundation. When the researchers heard money they talked to me."

A year after the ordeal, Charlotte met a friend whose mother also succumbed to cancer of the ovaries. The friend's mother was operated on and, like Charlotte's mother, was closed up without resection of the diseased parts. Her cancer was likewise too far gone. The friend blindly trusted the doctor's advice, which was to do nothing—not even conventional chemotherapy. And wouldn't you know, the friend's mother lived as long as Charlotte's.

The moral of this story is that when you're rolling against the Big Casino, you may not need all the help you can get—if you're lucky enough to get it in the first place.

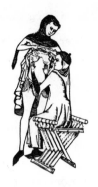

CHAPTER ELEVEN

Cancer Is Better Than Ever–in Hollywood

Cancer may be the second leading cause of death in the United States, but can it act? Until recently, Hollywood wouldn't touch the disease with a ten-foot balance sheet. It was much more aesthetic to eliminate sickly characters with old reliables like heart attack or tuberculosis. No muss, no fuss. How often did we see Edward G. Robinson clutch his chest and keel over for a fast exit? If the poor soul who was about to die had to hang on a while for dramatic purpose, then a trip to the TB sanatorium worked rather neatly. Willian Bendix could hardly avoid dying of throat cancer in *The Babe Ruth Story*, but the pathology of the Babe's illness struck out on film.

Love Story and *Brian's Song* finally cured Hollywood's fear of cancer. Ali MacGraw as the doomed Jennifer Cavilleri of Erich Segal's lachrymose script and James Caan as the ill-fated Chicago Bears fullback Brian Piccolo made metastasis safe for the screen. Tumors are now big entertainment. They have performed leading roles in *Bang the Drum Slowly*, several made for TV movies and various medical and nonmedical series.

For example, cancer played a double header on television one evening in the 1973 season when both *Marcus Welby, M.D.* (ABC) and *Police Story* (NBC) rolled out the terminal *deus ex machina*. Dr. Welby spread his usual balm over a cancer-ridden father who had lost his will to live. (On an earlier show Dr. Welby encouraged a rookie baseball player to coach the neighborhood kids while waiting for his brain tumor to send him to the eternal showers.) Meantime, *Police Story* was milking the disease with a new twist. Tensions were breaking up the veteran detective team of Paul Burke and Claude Akins. The burly Akins was behaving very strangely. His ten-year partner Burke couldn't figure out what was wrong. Eventually, Akins stupidly rushed a group of cornered gunmen instead of lying back until the reinforcements arrived. Naturally, the bad guys drilled him full of holes while Burke looked on helplessly. In the next scene the captain informs him that his buddy had advanced cancer. Suddenly, Burke gets the picture. When a cop dies on the job, it's double indemnity. If Akins was a dead man anyway, why shouldn't he arrange a killing—financial and otherwise—as long as nobody got hurt but himself and the taxpayers?

Kamikaze cancer had a subsequent run on *Kojak* when Harry Guardino, one of Telly Savalas' detectives, blackmailed a mobster into an unconstitutional shootout. Although Guardino had been popping painkillers during the hour, we did not learn his secret until after emergency surgery was performed. The bullets in Guardino's chest were removed, said the long-faced surgeon, but he couldn't get all the cancer out.

What if a young Idaho schoolteacher thought she was dying of leukemia and therefore decided to live it up in San Francisco until death called? Say she becomes bored in a fancy Fairmont Hotel suite and arranges a contract for her own assassination by an unknown hit man who is free to strike any time. Then a routine check-up, by a San Francisco doctor reveals that her fatal leukemia was actually a harmless bout of mononucleosis. Of course, she would rather not be murdered for mono. You could build an entire movie around the police's attempt to locate the hired mercy killer. The story is too incredible, right? Not if you've seen the CBS TV-film *The Face of Fear*, starring Ricardo Montalban as the exasperated cop and Elizabeth Ashley as the scatterbrained schoolteacher. Only in Hollywood is cancer better than ever.

Despite the exploitative nature of most media malignancy, blacklisting gains nothing. Ignorance is a poor poultice. But so is romanticizing the disease. Nobody with chronic leukemia goes out with the kind of apple-cheeked spunk Ali MacGraw exhibited on her deathbed in *Love Story*. And no young girl ever beat lymphoma with just a few shots of her boyfriend's blood—as Season Hubley did with a little intravenous help from Desi Arnez, Jr., in the 1973 ABC-TV movie *She Lives*.

Brian's Song, an earlier ABC-TV film, should retire the trophy for the worst cancer rip-off in any medium. Based on a chapter from Gale Sayers' autobiography—*I Am Third*—the screenplay emphasized the interracial friendship between two Chicago Bears teammates. Sayers (Billie Dee Williams) was the star fullback and Brian Piccolo (James Caan) his white substitute. And cancer the *deus ex machina*.

The movie opens with a voiceover: "Ernest Hemingway said that every true story ends in death. Well this *is* a true story." Hemingway was only partly right. Even phony stories end in death and *Brian's Song* is one of them.

The brotherhood plot derives from the Bears' decision to integrate their rooming on the road. Piccolo and Sayers were the first pair selected to break the team's color line. In the film this portentous event occurs in training camp during their rookie season in

1965. J.C. Caroline, apparently an assistant coach and a black himself, socks it to Sayers in the presence of Coach George Halas and Bears Vice-President Ed Mc-Caskey. "You're going to be called a Tom by some blacks and an uppity nigger by some whites. . . . You're going to rock the boat, Sayers—and there's plenty of people around who are already seasick." Piccolo is then surprised when he finds Sayers in his room because nobody told him of the arrangement. Anyway the two become instant soul brothers on and off the field. Black and white together, with a musical lift from Michel Legrand, who also provided the score for *Love Story*.

Writer William Blinn, who cut short his Emmy acceptance speech pleading that he had to go to the john, was accurate about Piccolo and Sayers rooming together. But everything else is fiction. They were neither bosom buddies nor roommates from the beginning. Contrary to *Brian's Song*, Piccolo didn't even make the team as a rookie. They hardly spoke to each other the first two years. After the forced integration in their third season, they still didn't see much of each other socially. Sayers admits this in his book. J. C. Caroline never coached Piccolo and Sayers on the Bears and couldn't have delivered his straight-from-the-shoulder speech. Actually Ed McCaskey did the honors. "I went to both fellows," he remarks, "and there was no drama to it at all. It was kind of a joke." The real closeness developed when cancer struck. Sayers, alone among the Bears players, would often fly half across the country to be with Piccolo during his illness. ("A lot of guys would have flown to Memorial Hospital in New York to see Brian if the team picked up the expenses," says a former Bear who suspects the company financed Sayers' corporate works of mercy.) But he was not Piccolo's best friend on the Bears—a fact Blinn carefully hid.

The Bears organization is understandably unhappy with the many distortions and inventions in the film. Coach Halas feels ABC was rather cheesy about the whole deal and to this day has not signed a release for his characterization. To the Bears' annoyance, Blinn called his own game. "He was not open to suggestions at any time," complains McCaskey.

Blinn was his own medicine man too, and so the cancer theme suffered from the same overdramatization. None of the doctors who treated Piccolo's chest tumor at Memorial Hospital was consulted. In the original script, Blinn had Piccolo's surgeon, Dr. Edward Beattie, brusquely inform him that a second operation would be necessary: "I know this is a bother at a time like this, Mr. Piccolo," Dr. Beattie's caricature stated, "but hospitals have their rules and regulations, you see, and I'll need your signature on this surgical consent for the operation." Dr. Beattie protested to the Bears. What was this nonsense? He performed three operations on Piccolo over several months and became emotionally involved in the case. He never talked to Piccolo or any patient like that. Joy Piccolo, Brian's wife, told *Brian's Song* director Buzz Kulik to change it. ABC kept the scene but substituted a hospital official for Dr. Beattie. Just like Ali MacGraw, James Caan went out like a dream while Williams and their wives choked up. (Actually, Mr. and Mrs. Sayers were a thousand miles distant when Piccolo expired.)

"I love you, Brian—I love you. . . ." Joy whispers.

"Who'd believe it, Joy—who'd ever believe it. . . . ." Brian barely responds and then peacefully passes away before us.

In truth, Piccolo's last words were screamed with tubes hanging out of him. "Can you believe it, Joy. Can you believe this shit?" he shouted to his wife in despair. Not enough blood was getting to the brain and Piccolo was alternatively delirious and agitated. Joy Piccolo asked Brian's doctor to quiet her husband down with a sedative and he never regained consciousness. Brian Piccolo died cold, clammy, and in shock, fifty pounds underweight, and gasping for breath as the tumor put the squeeze on his heart.

Why did the American Cancer Society, which should know better, give *Brian's Song* a citation? "We understood it was fictional," a spokesman explains, "but we're trying to get people into the doctor's office early. If you portray cancer on that screen with all its degradation and pain, you haven't a prayer. If they ever walked into a cancer ward, they'd run away so fast. And we want them to stop running away from this goddamn disease."

In the Hollywood dream factory, cancer is never having to say, "Can you believe this shit?"

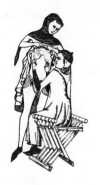

CHAPTER TWELVE

Cancer Politics

By all that's good and holy, cancer ought to be above politics. The final version of the National Cancer Act of 1971 passed both houses of Congress without a dissenting vote, and the once veto-happy President Nixon eagerly signed the bill. As the right disease in the right place at the right time, cancer apparently faces a united opposition.

In reality, the politics of cancer has been a whited sepulchre. Despite the professed purity of motives on every side, the National Cancer Act was one of the hardest and dirtiest fought pieces of legislation in the 92nd Congress. It pitted the White House against the Democratic party's most appealing presidential candidate, flushed out the worst instincts of Washington's health bureaucrats, sullied the unblemished record of the American Cancer Society lobby and turned medical brother against brother. Malignancy makes for estranged bedfellows. Few participants emerged from this chamber-room brawl unscathed. How could it have been otherwise when the primary issue seemed not the cure for cancer but rather the power, money, and prestige that the act would apportion?

Even passage did not bring peace. In 1973, Dr. Charles C. Edwards, assistant secretary of the Department of Health, Education and Welfare for health, would call the act an administrative "mistake." The scientific community, in turn, would resent the Nixon administration's meddling with established research procedures to save a buck in the budget. Before the war on cancer was three years old, the generals would be confused and the troops demoralized.

What sort of organization would lead the stepped-up assault on cancer?—that was the original question—whether it was wiser for the National Cancer Institite to remain under the wing of the Department of Health, Education, and Welfare and the National Institutes of Health or become a separate agency of the government reporting directly to the President. On one side, the cancer lobby and the overwhelming majority of the Senate declared for a totally independent agency (like the Manhattan Project and Apollo Program), which would be liberated from the bureaucratic oppression of HEW and NIH. On the other side, med school deans, scores of medical associations, and the House of Representatives warned against fragmenting biomedical research by snatching NCI from its natural habitat within HEW and NIH.

There were five principals in the struggle to pass cancer legislation in 1971:

President Richard Nixon—Before the billion dollar cancer ball started rolling on Capitol Hill, the Nixon administration was asking for substantial cuts in 1970 House-approved research funds. Furthermore, Nixon's position on cancer legislation changed four times in 1971. But when the dust settled he snagged all the credit. "It was the hottest goddamn thing in Washington and Nixon just got on the teat," states the administrative assistant of a leading Democratic congressman.

Senator Edward M. Kennedy—As chairman of the Senate Health Subcommittee, Kennedy introduced the independence-minded conquest of cancer bill (later known as the National Cancer Act), which he inherited from his predecessor, Senator Ralph Yarborough. He let the President steal the show but the script was largely his own. The "Kennedy" bill passed the Senate 79-1.

Mrs. Mary Lasker—Through the Albert and Mary Lasker Foundation, this philanthropist has given away tons of cash for medical causes since 1942. A formidable lobbyist in her fashion, she is honorary chairman of the American Cancer Society's Board of Directors and allegedly a secret sponsor of an expensive newspaper ad campaign calculated to embarrass congressmen who wouldn't take the proper line on the cancer bill.

Benno Schmidt—He is cancer's Kissinger. Schmidt, the managing partner of the venture capital firm of J.H. Whitney & Co., chaired a committee of consultants for Senator Yarborough in 1970. The can-do recommendations of this committee formed the rationale for the government's great leap forward in cancer funding. Schmidt acted as a valuable go-between when the White House and the Senate were negotiating their differences. After the passage of the Act, Nixon appointed him chairman of the three-man President's Cancer Panel which oversees NCI's National Cancer Program and reports directly to the President. And he's retaining this post under President Ford.

Representative Paul Rogers—*Medical World News* refers to Rogers, chairman of the House Subcommittee on Public Health and Environment, as "health's new strong man in Congress." That he is. He despised the idea of separating the National Cancer Institute from the National Institutes of Health. The Rogers cancer bill retained the integrity of the latter and passed the House 350-5.

How the National Cancer Act eventually prospered

is a long and complicated story which will be rendered here short and simple.

To the best of former Senator Yarborough's recollection, he first had the notion of a grand-scale drive on cancer in 1960 or thereabouts. While sitting on the Health Subcommittee he heard Dr. Rhee Clark of Houston's M.D. Anderson Hospital and Tumor Clinic testify that a billion dollars a year for ten years would cure about 90 percent of cancer. When he succeeded to the chairmanship of the Senate Committee on Labor and Public Welfare in 1969, he had the pick of any subcommittee chairmanship as well. "I chose Health so I could push this thing," he says. He solicited Mrs. Lasker's advice on the best way to proceed in arousing Congress, which is not notorious for billion-dollar bonanzas in medicine. (However, our elected officials have come a fair distance since 1927, the year they ignored the first piece of cancer legislation but managed to appropriate $10 million to rid the heartland of the insatiate corn borer.) Lasker suggested the expert-panel route with her friend Benno Schmidt as its prime mover. Yarborough didn't expect Schmidt would be available. After all, he is a director of twenty-five business enterprises with holdings in the United States, Australia, New Zealand, Western Europe, and Africa. But as chairman of the board of Memorial Hospital, Schmidt has a soft spot for cancer. He enlisted in Yarborough's project in the spring of 1970 and later that fall delivered the panel's report. The government's health bureaucracy was criticized as cumbersome and unfit for an effective war on cancer: "Obviously, from many standpoints it can be argued that any cancer program should be in the Department of Health, Education, and Welfare and indeed that it should be in the National Institutes of Health. However, there is real doubt whether the kind of organization that is required for this program can in fact be achieved within the National Institutes of Health or within the Department of Health, Education, and Welfare. Apart from the question of whether it can be done, there is also the question of whether it would be wise to require the Secretary of Health, Education, and Welfare to attempt to give cancer the priority necessary to carry out the congressional mandate ("the conquest of cancer is a national crusade") in a department charged with the multiple health and other responsibilities of that Department."

Schmidt's executive sense was offended by the HEW-NIH modus operandi, whereby the director of NCI reported to the deputy director of NIH, who reported to the surgeon general, who reported to an assistant secretary of HEW, who reported to the undersecretary of HEW, who reported to the secretary. "We looked at the situation to see how the layering worked," he would later remark, "and we found that it works to bring about inordinate delays; so far there has been no comprehensive overall program plan. There is no clearly defined authority and responsibility." Schmidt and his panel of experts concluded that cancer deserved nothing less than an institute free and clear of bureaucratic entanglements.

Senator Yarborough was defeated for a third term in November, 1970. Senator Edward Kennedy assumed the chairmanship of the subcommittee and shepherded Yarborough's original bill (which embodied Schmidt's recommendations) through hearings in March of 1971. After listening to objections from the HEW-NIH complex and the Association of American Medical Schools (which feared that a separate cancer agency would drain federal funds from medical schools), the subcommittee still bought the cancer lobby's concept of independence, although certain concessions were allowed. NCI would stay nominally within NIH, but would be permitted a separate budget and the privilege to report to the President.

The Nixon administration realized the game was up. If it couldn't beat Kennedy, it would have to join him. So on May 11, the very day the subcommittee was to mark up its bill, S. 34, President Nixon issued a statement paralleling the Senate's provisions and had former Senator Peter Dominick (R., Colo.) introduce S. 1828, the White House bill. "We kept telling them" a Dominick aide candidly admitted, "that the only way to effectively oppose Kennedy's bill was with another bill. The Senate is a legislative body. When it became clear that S. 34 would sail through committee and the Senate, that there was no stopping it, the administration introduced a bill." Curiously, the Nixon statement and the Nixon bill didn't jibe. It was suspected that HEW bureaucrats had sabotaged the wording of the presidential statement in a last-ditch effort to save NIH from potentially disastrous vivisection.

Then a splendid deal was arranged. Nixon wanted publicity and Kennedy wanted a cancer bill. So Kennedy offered to approve Nixon's S. 1828 as long as the language was substantially that of his own S. 34. The President bit, and the bipartisan S. 1828 passed the Senate easily on July 7. Only Senator Gaylord Nelson of Wisconsin voted no, dismissing the affair as "a mischievous political compromise of a very important scientific matter."

The Nixon-Kennedy bill should have been a cinch in the House. But Representative Paul Rogers had other plans. He revived the anti-independence argument in September and October hearings, insisting that the S. 1828 had not satisfactorily solved the problem of NCI status. It was "within" NIH but its budget and chain of command were completely outside. Rogers counterattacked with H.R. 10681, which elevated the director of NCI to associate director of NIH and permitted the secretary of HEW and director of NIH to "comment" on NCI's autonomous budget. A three-man President's panel would also be established to serve as the White House's watchdog.

Which bill did Nixon prefer? He said he liked them both and either would be acceptable. This was his fourth modification on cancer. First, he was opposed to any new legislation; second, he put forth his own bill; third, he supported the Kennedy bill in the guise of his own; and then he favored the Senate and House bills simultaneously. Not for nothing did they call him tricky.

Actually, S. 1828 and H.R. 10681 weren't too far apart. The two sides reconciled their differences and forged a bill much superior to the original proposals. NCI was granted independence within the framework of NIH; its budget couldn't be tampered with but HEW and NIH could add obiter dicta; and the President's panel would assure a hearing at the White House. Congress was happy and the President was even happier because the National Cancer Act of 1971 had his number (S. 1828) on it. "I must say the compromise worked out pretty well," confesses Benno Schmidt, who initially stumped for absolute autonomy. "I would not even go back to the original legislation."

The act generously authorized $400 million for fiscal 1972, $500 million for fiscal 1973, and $600 million for fiscal 1974. With that kind of money NCI was mandated to get a coordinated National Cancer Program on the road. But despite the President's promises, executive penny-pinching prevented NCI from going full tilt. For three consecutive years, the Office of Management and Budget shortchanged the cancer effort. In 1972, NCI received $378.6 million (plus $42 million for cancer control); in 1973, $431.2 million after $60 million was impounded; and in fiscal 1974, $589.15 million including the $60 million previously impounded. That's about $100 million less than the total commitment Nixon had grandiosely announced. On top of the lower spending his administration cut off all NIH pre- and post-doctoral training grants in January of 1973. This budgetary move meant that young researchers, including prospective cancer specialists, would no longer be subsidized during their extended scientific apprenticeships. "How can the President declare a crusade against cancer," asked Dr. Giulio J. D'Angio, chairman of Memorial Hospital's Diagnostic Radiation Department, "and then decimate the troops?"

Nobel Laureate Salvatore Luria, director of MIT's Cancer Center, has an explanation. "The people appointed to top positions in government agencies today are more likely to be the kind of individuals who don't really understand the subtle points of a purely intellectual enterprise like research. So I wouldn't be surprised if the Office of Management and Budget officials were know-nothing individuals who feel that anything that doesn't bring results within twelve months and a cure within two years is wasted money."

Columbia University virologist Sol Spiegelman seconds Luria's contempt for health bureaucrats. "I don't think these people would have supported Fleming's research on penicillin," he says. "They wouldn't have given Fleming a penny because they couldn't have foreseen what came out of that sort of research."

What does Caspar Weinberger, formerly of OMB (of all places) and later secretary of HEW, answer? Just what you would expect. "If you don't care about inflation," he remarked on CBS's *Sixty Minutes* in 1974, "if you don't care about tax increases, which was the case during the mid-sixties then any increase request is granted and everybody keeps level of criticism quite low. But we felt it was essential to try to do something about getting at one of the major root causes of inflation—which is government spending."

It is hardly comforting to realize that the secretary of Health, Education, and Welfare worried more about inflation than the cure of cancer.

Despite the executive branch's clumsy and unvisionary attempt to rein the stampede against cancer, prospects are improving. In the spring of 1974, Congress passed the National Research Training Act, which reinstated the concept of pre- and post-doctoral research support. Last year Congress also renewed the National Cancer Act for three years. The National Cancer Advisory Board has requested $750 million for fiscal 1975. The final appropriation is expected to be between $690 and $710 million. (Plus $53.5 million for cancer control.) In addition, Congress has authorized $830 million (plus $68.5 million for cancer control) for fiscal 1976 and $985 million (plus $88.5 million for cancer control) for 1977. These greatly expanded budgets assure NCI of at least two billion dollars more in a very short time.

Even if the President were totally incontinent with cancer funding and NCI could mint money, there are those who believe its National Cancer Program—the new name for NCI's coordination of all cancer-related activities within NIH—still wouldn't hit the jackpot. There is a crisis in confidence among cancer researchers. Many of them consider NCI Big Brother and the National Cancer Program Plan—a detailed, step-by-step strategy of cancer priorities leading to the final solution—a systems analysis fiasco.

For example, in the view of Dr. James D. Watson, whose professional achievement and three-year membership (1972–1974) on the twenty-two-man National Cancer Advisory Board qualify him to comment, the National Cancer Program is all wrong. In 1953 Dr. Watson, then 25, and his colleague Dr. Francis Crick announced the discovery of the structure of DNA, the elusive hereditary molecule, at Cambridge University. Everybody talked about genes but nobody knew what they looked like before Watson and Crick figured out their double helix shape in one of the great scientific breakthroughs of the century. This development won them a Nobel Prize and cleared the trail for further probes into genetic material where the little C gets its big start. So even if Watson doesn't have a hand in the final understanding of why normal cells go awry, the fellows who do will probably be standing on his shoulders. That time could be rather far off, according to Watson, if we have to depend on the

National Cancer Program. "It's a bunch of shit," he says. "That plan isn't going to do any good."

One should not be taken aback by such plain-speaking because Watson is legendary for calling them as he sees them. *The Double Helix,* his inside account of the kicking and scratching behind the race to penetrate the mysterious DNA, so scandalized Harvard University Press that they turned the manuscript down and let another publishing house rake in its best-selling profits. "Like all good memoirs," Nobel Laureate P. B. Medewar commented in a review, "it has not been emasculated by considerations of good taste." And neither, it is clear, has a spot on the National Cancer Advisory Board dimmed Watson's desire for brutal frankness.

Dr. Watson divides his time between teaching molecular biology at Harvard and directing research at the Cold Spring Harbor Laboratory on Long Island, where I interrupted him one frozen winter weekend. He was sitting behind a slab desk in his neat harborside cottage office revising proofs of a book on tumor viruses. The Watson of middle age resembles the British character actor Alistair Sim (*The Lavender Hill Mob*). The overall similarity is uncanny—right down to the honks and wheezes of speech. Like Sim in his con man roles, Watson seems to enjoy trafficking in the outré. He grins a lot, especially on the subject of NCI's step-by-step outline for doing cancer in.

Does Watson suggest that the conquest of cancer can't be charted at all? "Not in the manner of the National Cancer Plan. That's a lot of crap," he remarks. "Yes, you can test for carcinogens, which is an experience in good organization. But you can't plan the conquest of cancer because you don't know what it is. You hope for unplanned observations." Can the 250 leading cancer specialists who put their heads together for four days in 1971 to devise the National Cancer Plan be wrong? "People who make discoveries don't go to those kinds of meetings," Watson replies without mercy. "People who do are usually long past the age of creativity. The plan was put together to impress Congress. Plus I think that Carl Baker [NCI director from 1969 to 1972] got a Master's degree in planning and loved flow diagrams."

It is Watson's impression that the new dollars didn't bring in any new ideas and that previously extant projects were simply increased proportionately. Therefore, he is positive money is being wasted at certain favored research institutes. "These places have reputations for mediocrity. I don't think they'd rank in the top forty in the country." Dr. Watson cites three well-known and lavishly supported cancer institutes: one is called "really lousy," a second "just awful" and a third "a semblance" of proficiency. (The public would be shocked to learn the targets of Watson's disesteem.) "Bob Good [president and director of the Sloan-Kettering Institute] offered very high salaries to at least three people I know and they haven't accepted. It's almost impossible to turn down a grant to M.D. Anderson because R. Lee Clark, director and surgeon-in-chief of M.D. Anderson Hospital, is on the President's Panel. Yet the best students will still go to Cal Tech, Stanford, Berkeley, and Harvard. And these places won't get any money to establish good programs, as students won't be interested in cancer."

Watson feels that tougher management at the top could turn things around. "NCI is very weak in strong people. Its situation is completely different from the Manhattan Project, which was full of scientists with strong academic careers behind them. The people in NCI, however, are not the best people in American science. They spend all their time putting out big books."

What ever happened to the National Cancer Advisory Board, which was mandated to "advise and assist the Director of the National Cancer Institute with respect to the National Cancer program"? Were Watson and his cohorts powerless to change this allegedly disastrous state of affairs? "The Board could function better if it were presented with choices," he replies. "We weren't asked to decide between two choices, but to approve something like the national colon program—it's down at M.D. Anderson. But every time we voted no, it was like voting against motherhood. On the whole, American science won't get any better by these parochial programs."

Watson jokes about one board meeting when they were briefed on the miracles of chemotherapy by NCI's Gordon Zubrod with the usual slides on leukemia, Burkitt's lymphoma, Hodgkins disease. Watson couldn't refrain from popping an embarrassing question about increased lifespan in the other 85 percent of cancers. "It's not that I don't respect Zubrod," he says. "It's just that you wonder whether you should be putting your eggs in other baskets. Of course, there was no answer. If they had the data they'd give it to you."

Apropos misallocation of resources Watson gives honorable mention to Dr. Sol Spiegelman, director of Columbia's Institute of Cancer Research. "The great white hope of NCI's Special Virus Cancer Program is Sol Spiegelman. He's a very intelligent and clever person, but he's also often wrong. Sol has the largest salary of any American virologist at $85,000. He thinks big and he's trying to find out what's up. Rauscher believes he's going to accomplish a lot. But Sol should be doing maybe 2 percent."

Presumably Watson has passed these observations on to the President's Panel Chairman Benno Schmidt. "He agrees with me, but he has conflicting pressures." Then what about Nixon himself? Surely a Nobel Laureate with his cancer credentials could have wangled a White House audience. "I think the man's a murderer," Watson said at the time, "I just won't talk to him. He's beyond the pale. I'll talk to Benno, but that's it."

When Dr. Watson talked, Benno Schmidt didn't listen very hard. "He was the most distinguished member of the cancer board," Schmidt remarks about the troublesome biologist, "but whether he was the best would be a matter of debate." The chairman of the President's Cancer Panel hardly conceals his contempt for Watson's criticism during a long conversation at his Rockefeller Center headquarters. Schmidt, sixty-four, looks like Walter Cronkite and similarly never raises his voice despite the harshness of his words.

"Dr. Watson has a high sense of excellence," Schmidt continues, "but he also has a high sense of his own opinion. Of course, I'm subject to conflicting pressures. I ought to be. And I try to recognize the validity of various viewpoints. Unfortunately, that's not Jim Watson. I don't agree with him that the National Cancer Plan is a lot of shit. He can't come to us and say: 'I don't know what I'm doing and neither do you, so give me my research money.' Watson's got to do on a small scale in his grant application exactly what he's criticizing on a large scale. I agree with Jim to the extent that the Plan should not be treated as an operation manual. But he wants to find the hundred brightest scientists and just hope for the best. I don't argue that the absence of a plan would be a disaster or mean that we'd be less likely to cure cancer without one. Rather, I contend that there is no better way to rub minds together than to bring in scientists from different fields to discuss and distill a problem. Cancer research is no more or no less circumscribed or uncircumscribed because of the existence of the Plan. Well, what good is it then? One of the obvious benefits, as I've said already, is group thinking. Another is that you gain an overall view that may be helpful in particular activities. The Plan may have caused stronger support for certain areas than was the case before the Plan. For example, (1) it brought into focus our neglect of immunology, and (2) on the clinical side, we were paying too little attention to the rehabilitation of the cancer patient."

Given the controversy that surrounds the National Cancer Institute and its Plan, how does Schmidt assess the progress his troops have made since the billion dollar plus National Cancer Act of 1971? "Naturally," he says, "I would have liked ten important discoveries. As far as the quality of administration—I've been in the Army, the State Department, and now this area of government activity, and in my judgment, the Cancer Program has been administered as well as I could expect any government program to be administered. Watson is wrong about the quality of NCI's directors. None has a Nobel Prize, but Doctors Rauscher, Zubrod, and Sanders are men of outstanding ability and dedication. They're also men of common sense. So it ill becomes Jim Watson to indulge in his propensity for smart aleckiness by reflecting on the performance of these men.

"The plain fact is that Dr. Watson is not impressed by anyone except himself. But he's entitled to be an egotist. He's done great things on this earth. I've said to him at a meeting, 'If you don't pay more attention to facts in the laboratory than you do here, then we ought to take a second look at the double helix.' "

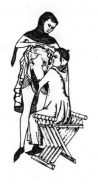

Epilogue

Dr. Edward Reich, the Rockefeller University researcher with an abhorrence for radical surgery, should have a little extra going for him in the lab. And wouldn't you know, he could have pulled it off. This genial middle-aged M.D.. who resembles the late Bennett Cerf, was gloriously close to a cure for cancer in 1973. Being a cautious man, he wouldn't make any predictions. He was only willing to remark that "it really is the kind of thing that people have always been looking for. Whether it turns out to be the answer or not is another story."

Dr. Reich's putative panacea appeared in January, 1973, in the *Journal of Experimental Medicine* under the title "An Enzymatic Function Associated with Transformation of Fibroblasts by Oncegenic Viruses." His paper recapitulated two years of investigation into the biochemical differences between normal and abnormal cells and now he thought he had a difference that could be fruitfully exploited. Talk about unplanned observations—Dr. Reich came across the big insight while reviewing the literature on cell transformation in 1966. He read that a Danish doctor by the name of A. Fischer noticed in the twenties that malignant tissues could lyse (or dissolve) plasma clots whereas normal cells could not. Unfortunately, Dr. Fischer never followed up this amazing development. To him the lysis was simply a nuisance because it interrupted his experiments. To Reich the lysis was the golden key. For clots don't lyse by themselves— this process depends on the activity of enzymes. Therefore, there had to be an enzymatic difference between normal and abnormal cells.

Reich was able to repeat Fischer's experiment in controlled cell cultures and discovered that the lysis was a rather general phenomenon in tissues made malignant by viruses and chemicals and in spontaneous human tumors. "The molecular analysis has proceeded quite a ways," he commented a short while after his article was published. "We know that the enzymatic activity which is called fibrinolysis is produced by the interaction of two factors—one in the serum and the other in the cell. Malignant tissues give rise to fibrinolysin on account of the cell factor. There seems to be no comparable factor in normal cells."

Terrific, but where does it get us? "There's a fair bit of clinical evidence," Reich resumes, "that tells us that the enzyme system must be at work in advanced malignant disease. What we're doing now is proceeding with the purification of the serum and cell factors with the idea of trying to use the information for diagnostic procedures and for providing a target for chemotherapy. There's even hope we may be able to apply some preventive measures if the enzyme system really turns out to be essential for the growth of tumors in animals. Although we know it's there, we're not quite positive it's indispensible to growth. All this is still in its infancy, but within the next year we ought to have a pretty clear view of things."

It is two years later and the view is apparently dim. Reich's breakthrough, like so many promising leads, hasn't broken through.

Cancer is still king and its reign assured for longer than we dare speculate. But when this disease is overthrown don't look to the news media for proof. The end to malignancy cannot be confirmed by an NCI press release, but rather by the gradual withering away of its metaphoric value. You will know cancer is dethroned when some future John Dean tells a future Richard Nixon that there is a heart attack growing on the presidency.

Philip Nobile is a contributing editor of *Esquire* and a nationally syndicated columnist. After taking graduate degrees in philosophy from Boston University and The University of Louvain (Belgium), he worked as an editor of *Commonweal* (1968–70) and began writing for several national publications including *The New York Review of Books* and *The New York Times Magazine.* He is the editor of *Catholic Nonsense, The New Eroticism, The Con III Controversy,* and *Favorite Movies* and co-editor of *The Berrigans* and *The Complete Ecology Fact Book.* He authored a 1973 book entitled, *Intellectual Skywriting.* Mr. Nobile was born and bred in Belmont, Massachusetts, and now lives on the upper tip of Manhattan with his wife Maureen and three young daughters Megan, Caitlin, and Maeve.

Date Due

FEB 25 '80	APR 22 1984	
	DEC 1 0 1984	
APR 4 80	APR 9 1986	
APR 17 '80	NOV 17 1987	
MAY 1 - 80	DEC 8 - 1987	
OCT 21 '80	FEB 23 1988	
DEC 1 '80	APR 5 1988	
12-18-80	DEC 1 4 1989	
FEB 17 '81	MAR 3 1991	
APR 12 '81		
5/8/8, CSP	MAY 1 9 1994	
DEC 8 - '81	FEB 2 8 1998	
OCT. -5 1982 -OCH, 82	APR 1 9 1999	
NOV 2 2 1982		
12-8-82		OCT 1 0 2002